# LIVER
# DETOX

# LIVER DETOX

## Cleansing through Diet, Herbs, and Massage

### CHRISTOPHER VASEY, N.D.

#### TRANSLATED BY JON E. GRAHAM

Healing Arts Press
Rochester, Vermont • Toronto, Canada

Healing Arts Press
One Park Street
Rochester, Vermont 05767
www.HealingArtsPress.com

Healing Arts Press is a division of Inner Traditions International

Originally published in French under the title *Je détoxique mon foie, c'est parti* by Éditions Jouvence, www.editions-jouvence.com, info@editions-jouvence.com
First U.S. edition published in 2018 by Healing Arts Press

*Note to the reader:* *This book is intended as an informational guide. The remedies, approaches, and techniques described herein are meant to supplement, and not to be a substitute for, professional medical care or treatment. They should not be used to treat a serious ailment without prior consultation with a qualified health care professional.*

**Library of Congress Cataloging-in-Publication Data**

Names: Vasey, Christopher, author.
Title: Liver detox : cleansing through diet, herbs, and massage / Christopher Vasey, N.D. ; translated by Jon E. Graham.
Other titles: Je détoxique mon foie, c'est parti. English
Description: Rochester, Vermont : Healing Arts Press, [2018] | Includes index.
Identifiers: LCCN 2017033321 (print) | LCCN 2017033859 (e-book) | ISBN 9781620556993 (pbk.) | ISBN 9781620557006 (e-book)
Subjects: LCSH: Liver—Popular works. | Diet therapy—Popular works. | Detoxification (Health)
Classification: LCC RC846 (e-book) | LCC RC846 .V3713 2018 (print) | DDC 616.3/620654—dc23
LC record available at https://lccn.loc.gov/2017033321

Printed and bound in the United States by Versa Press, Inc.

10  9  8  7  6  5  4  3  2  1

Text design and layout by Virginia Scott Bowman
This book was typeset in Garamond Premier Pro, Gill Sans, and Avenir with Raleway, Leawood, and Hypatia Sans used as display typefaces
Illustrations by Rosalie Vasey

To send correspondence to the author of this book, mail a first-class letter to the author c/o Inner Traditions • Bear & Company, One Park Street, Rochester, VT 05767, and we will forward the communication, or contact the author directly at **www.christophervasey.ch/anglais/home.html**.

# CONTENTS

## PART 1
. . . . . . . . . . .
### *Understanding the Liver and How It Works*

## PART 2
··········
### *How to Detoxify Your Liver*

# HOW WELL DOES YOUR LIVER FUNCTION?

## A Self-Diagnosis Checklist

Most of us don't have a very clear idea of where the liver is located in our bodies, never mind what roles it plays in our bodily functions. Indigestion? Bad breath? It's a common misconception that these and other symptoms are rooted in the stomach or intestines, and it's equally common to believe that some kind of prescription or over-the-counter medication will fix them. Sure, you can drink a fizzy tablet dissolved in water and feel better in the short term, but to truly restore your body to health, you'll need to look to the liver.

A good place to start is to evaluate how well your liver is functioning right now:

| | | |
|---|---|---|
| I regularly experience digestive problems. | ☐ Yes | ☐ No |
| Eggs or pastries make me feel nauseous. | ☐ Yes | ☐ No |
| I tend to get drowsy after a meal. | ☐ Yes | ☐ No |
| My tongue is often coated when I wake up in the morning. | ☐ Yes | ☐ No |
| I often have bad breath. | ☐ Yes | ☐ No |
| I regularly experience gas and bloating. | ☐ Yes | ☐ No |
| I'm often constipated. | ☐ Yes | ☐ No |

| | | |
|---|---|---|
| I have hemorrhoids. | ☐ Yes | ☐ No |
| The whites of my eyes have a yellowish cast. | ☐ Yes | ☐ No |
| I feel tired and low energy all day long. | ☐ Yes | ☐ No |
| I get headaches on a regular basis. | ☐ Yes | ☐ No |
| I get hives when I overeat. | ☐ Yes | ☐ No |
| I like large meals. | ☐ Yes | ☐ No |
| I often eat fried foods or dishes with sauce or gravy. | ☐ Yes | ☐ No |
| I drink alcohol on a regular basis. | ☐ Yes | ☐ No |
| I smoke tobacco. | ☐ Yes | ☐ No |

### Analysis of the Answers

*If you have no more than two "yes" answers,* your liver is most likely functioning well, but there are many useful things this book can teach you in order to keep it in optimal working order.

*Three to five "yes" answers* indicate that your liver has trouble performing its job, and steps should be taken to detoxify it.

*If you have more than six "yes" answers,* these are not healthy conditions. Your liver is overburdened and it would be smart to detoxify it as soon as you are able.

---

### ⚠ Caution!

Liver diseases that are not treated properly can have serious consequences for your health. The advice and recommendations provided in this book are not intended to replace the care and treatment of a skilled medical practitioner. If you are not sure about something, or if your condition is serious, please seek prompt medical attention.

---

# THE IMPORTANCE OF A HEALTHY LIVER

*I regularly suffer from digestive problems. I do not seem to be able to eat a number of foods without discomfort. I feel heavy and often experience stomach pains, as well as headaches. I often feel tired and lack enthusiasm. Furthermore, I have acne and I'm often constipated . . .*

Stop! How long are you going to tolerate these problems? You may believe they are inevitable and there is nothing you can do about them, but they are all only symptoms of an overtaxed liver. By cleansing and detoxifying your liver, eliminating all the wastes, fats, and toxins that overburden it, you will regenerate it. This will allow you to get rid of all those tedious problems and you will recover both your health and vitality.

Physical health depends on the good functioning of *all* the body's organs. When just one of these organs becomes weak, the entire body suffers. Although each and every organ is vitally important, the liver is particularly crucial since it clears the way for the other organs to do their jobs. It is the first line of defense in confronting toxins and toxic substances that enter the organism from outside, which makes it the primary defender and protector of the body.

When the liver is unable to perform its given task, the organic cellular terrain becomes increasingly saturated with unwanted substances. According to the principles of natural medicine, this collection of harmful substances is the starting point for the vast majority of our diseases, because the body is under attack and therefore prevented from functioning properly.

We live in a culture that promotes overeating, overmedication, and widespread consumption of stimulants. We also have significant amounts of environmental pollution coming from our air, water, pesticides in our food, and toxic substances in everyday products that have become nearly impossible to avoid. All of these elements place a heavy demand upon the liver, causing it to become congested with wastes. The difficulty the liver experiences dealing with the mass of toxins and toxic substances assaulting it can be directly linked to the increase in cardiovascular, allergic, and immune system disorders we see so often today. When we support and detoxify the liver, we allow it to regenerate, which in turn gives protection to the entire body.

In most people the liver is overworked, weakened, and, quite frankly, diseased. While this book is addressed to those individuals suffering from digestive disorders linked to the liver, it also and just as importantly speaks to all those suffering from other diseases who are aware of the pivotal role the liver can play in restoring health.

The first part of this book explains the importance of detoxification for recovering your health by touching on the key notions of terrain, toxins, eliminatory organs and their functions, and draining. Once you are more aware of what the liver does, it may be easier to understand the importance of its efficiency. Poor liver function has many dire consequences that can become quite serious over time. As liver dysfunction is essentially due to the congestion of the organ by toxins, treatment primarily consists of detoxification. The second part of this book presents various ways to detoxify that are effective, efficient, and easy to apply. At the end of this section you will also find effective home remedies and treatments. They are simple enough for everyone to follow, but if you have any doubts or questions, always consult a medical professional.

## TEST YOUR LIVER IQ

1. Is the liver only a digestive organ?    ☐ Yes    ☐ No
2. How many functions do you think the liver performs?    ☐ 1    ☐ 48    ☐ 500
3. What percentage of imbibed alcohol is neutralized by the liver?    ☐ 15%    ☐ 50%    ☐ 95%
4. Does the liver eliminate toxins in bile?    ☐ Yes    ☐ No
5. How many liters of bile does the liver produce daily?    ☐ 0.2    ☐ 0.5    ☐ 1
6. Can the liver kill germs?    ☐ Yes    ☐ No
7. Is liver function stimulated by heat?    ☐ Yes    ☐ No
8. Is tobacco harmful to the liver?    ☐ Yes    ☐ No
9. Is the liver capable of neutralizing poisons?    ☐ Yes    ☐ No
10. Does eating fats fatigue the liver?    ☐ Yes    ☐ No
11. Do medicinal plants stimulate liver function?    ☐ Yes    ☐ No
12. Does the liver have any influence on glycemia?    ☐ Yes    ☐ No

### Answers

1. No. 2. 500. 3. 95%. 4. Yes. 5. 1 liter. 6. Yes. 7. Yes. 8. Yes. 9. Yes. 10. Yes. 11. Yes. 12. Yes.

### *Analysis of the Answers*

*Up to four correct answers:* You don't know very much about the liver, but this book will help you learn more.

*From five to eight correct answers:* You have some good information about the liver, but it's a complex organ and there's more for you to learn here.

*From nine to twelve correct answers:* Bravo, you already know a great deal and you can use this book to help you fill in any missing elements.

---

### ☝ Good to Know

Strictly speaking, the word *toxin* should only be used to refer to wastes produced by the body. Poisons that enter the organism from outside (the heavy metals of chemical pollution, for example) are designated by the adjective *toxic*.

In everyday speech, however, and for the purpose of simplification, the word *toxin* is also used in a general sense to designate all substances that can cause harm to the body, both toxins and toxic substances.

For ease of understanding, I will use *toxin* in the broader sense in this book, and only use the word *toxic* when it specifically and exclusively concerns toxic substances, or when necessary to prove a point.

---

# PART 1

······

*Understanding
the Liver
and How It Works*

# 1

# WHY DETOXIFY
# YOUR LIVER?

The detoxification of the body overall, and of the liver in particular, is of the highest importance in naturopathy. The value of this therapeutic procedure will be more apparent when you have become acquainted with the notion of the terrain—the body's cellular environment—as it is explained in natural medicine.

---

### ? Did You Know?

Naturopathy is a unique field of noninvasive primary health care that emphasizes health maintenance, prevention, and self-healing using methods and substances that encourage the body to heal itself.

---

## THE CONCEPT OF TERRAIN

Your body is a collection of cells, and your organs are clusters of cells. A cell is the basic unit of structure in every living thing. Cells in turn contain specialized interior structures called *organelles,* which have specific responsibilities for producing materials used elsewhere within the cell or in the body. Their activity ultimately enables the body to breathe, produce energy, eliminate wastes, reproduce, and send and receive messages.

---

### ? Did You Know?

Cells are all constructed in the same basic model but differ from each other based on their function. This is how we make distinctions among kidney, liver, intestine, bone, muscle, and nerve cells, as well as red and white blood cells, ova, spermatozoa, and so on.

---

Like every living thing, cells can survive only in a favorable environment. In the human body this environment is liquid and represents 70 percent of our body weight, forming what we call its *terrain*. The terrain encompasses various fluids.

Some of these fluids are in direct contact with the cells:

♦ *Intracellular fluid* has been given this name because it fills the interior of the cells. Our physical organism is composed primarily of this fluid, which represents 50 percent of our body weight.

♦ *Extracellular fluid,* or *interstitial fluid,* is outside the cells—that is, in the spaces between them. It bathes and surrounds the cells. Extracellular fluid forms the direct external environment of the cell and represents 15 percent of our body weight.

The other terrain fluids are not in direct contact with the cells:

- *Blood* circulates in the blood vessels.
- *Lymph* travels through the lymphatic vessels.

Combined, these last two fluids represent 5 percent of our body weight.

---

### ? **Did You Know?**

Only 30 percent of body weight consists of solid particles, which are primarily mineral salts: calcium, magnesium, potassium, and so on. The highest concentrations of solid particles are found in the skeleton, skull, hair, and tendons. Mineral salts also play a part in the composition of cell walls, tissues, and organs.

---

Because a cell's survival is entirely dependent upon the environment in which it is located, the composition of these bodily fluids is of critical importance.

## IDEAL TERRAIN

There is an ideal composition of the terrain that provides vitality and maximum stamina to the cells and organs for optimal physical health. A fundamental consequence of this desirable state of affairs is that any modification of this composition compromises your health and makes you vulnerable to illness.*

Changes in the composition of the body's cellular terrain occur primarily because of substances that have been added to its ideal state. These are substances that either are not for-

---

*For more information about maintaining optimal terrain, see my book *The Naturopathic Way: How to Detox, Find Quality Nutrition, and Restore Your Acid-Alkaline Balance* (Healing Arts Press, 2009).

eign to the terrain but are normally present in smaller quantities (uric acid, urea, and so forth) or substances that normally do not enter into the composition of the terrain (pollutants, food additives, and so forth). This accumulation of toxins that overburden the terrain is, according to natural medicine, a profound cause of disease. The root problem here is excess, and healing requires elimination of these toxins.

The terrain can also be altered by the absence of substances necessary for its ideal composition. These are substances such as vitamins, minerals, and trace elements that are normally present in the terrain but, for one reason or another, are temporarily not present in sufficient quantities. The root problem here is deficiency, which can be treated by supplying the body the nutrients it is lacking, through either diet or supplements.

## HOW TOXINS MAKE US SICK

When toxins collect in the body, they can make us sick in a number of ways.

The blood becomes thicker, and because it is now denser and heavier, it can no longer circulate easily through the blood vessels. Wastes that normally would be transported to the excretory organs by the bloodstream enter the lymph and other cellular fluids. The longer this contaminated and congested state lasts, the more corrupted these fluids will be.

Over time, the cells can find themselves bathing in a veritable swamp, the inert mass of which paralyzes all exchanges. Supplies of oxygen and nutrients can no longer make their way to the cells, so cells can not accomplish their work anymore, nor can the organs they constitute. Wastes accumulate, which reduces the body's ability to function properly.

The walls of the blood vessels become carpeted with wastes, reducing their diameter and slowing circulation, which in turn has an adverse effect on tissue irrigation and exchange.

The joints become blocked, the kidneys become clogged and eliminate wastes much less effectively, the skin closes up, and the liver becomes congested.

The body's tissues and mucous membranes are irritated by wastes. They become inflamed and over the long term become hardened and sclerotic. They also become more prone to infections. Harmful cellular mutations (cancer) begin to occur.

The harmful effects of toxins are due to:

- *Their mass.* They take up so much space that they hinder and block the vessels and cells.
- *Their aggressiveness.* They irritate, inflame, and destroy cells.

## ILLNESS CAUSED
## BY AN OVERLOAD OF TOXINS

It is logical to conclude that toxins are the basic factor in the onset of disease, and this can, in fact, be observed quite easily. When faced with an accumulation of toxins, the body does not remain passive but actively seeks to rid itself of them. Illnesses are therefore due both to the damage brought about by the presence of toxins and to the attempts of the body to expel the toxins.

For example, in respiratory illnesses we sneeze, cough, or expectorate to get rid of substances that are overloading the alveoli (asthma), bronchia (bronchitis), throat (coughs), sinuses (sinusitis), or nose (common cold).

All skin disorders are due to the rejection of either acidic substances by the sudoriferous glands (dry eczema, cracked and chapped skin) or colloidal wastes by the sebaceous glands (acne, boils, greasy skin, oozing eczema).

The presence of excess food substances in the stomach and intestines can cause regurgitation, indigestion, nausea, vomiting, or diarrhea. When these substances are irritating or fermenting, they cause inflammation of the mucous membranes of the digestive tract (gastritis, enteritis, colitis) or they produce gas (bloating).

---

### ⚠ Caution!

Intestinal fermentation and putrefaction produce toxic and irritating substances such as indole, phenol, hydrogen sulfite, methane, and ptomaine, which attack and inflame the mucous membranes of the intestine.

---

Joints become inflamed, blocked, and painful, and unless treated, they may become severely deformed (rheumatoid arthritis). In the case of gout, sharp, needlelike "crystals" of uric acid deposit may form in a joint or surrounding tissue, causing inflammation and tissue damage.

Cardiovascular diseases are due to the presence of surplus substances (cholesterol, fatty acids) that thicken the blood, accumulate in the arteries and thicken the walls (arteriosclerosis), and inflame the walls of blood vessels (phlebitis), which can either deform them (varicose veins) or clog them (heart attack, stroke, embolism).

In renal (kidney) disease, the culprit substances are protein wastes. In the case of obesity, it is fat. In diabetes, the culprit is sugar. Carcinogenic substances are at fault in cancer, as are allergens in allergies. The toxic agent in stomach ulcers is gastric acid.

> *Health results from finding a balance between the*
> *production and elimination of toxins and waste.*
> ROBERT MASSON, FOUNDER OF CENA, THE
> EUROPEAN CENTER FOR APPLIED NATUROPATHY

## WHAT IS THE SOURCE OF TOXINS?

Some toxins present in the body come from wear and tear of the tissues. The body must continually eliminate the remnants of depleted cells, the corpses of red blood cells, used mineral salts, carbon dioxide, ammonia, and so forth. The vast majority of toxins come from the use of food substances by the body. Proteins create uric acid and urea, glucose produces lactic acid, and fats create a variety of acids and cholesterol.

The production of these toxins is normal and the body is equipped to eliminate them.

In the event of overeating, however, the level of toxins increases far beyond what is considered to be normal. Consequently, in industrialized societies where overeating is common, the body takes in and produces an abnormal amount of toxins, which eventually will exceed the body's capacity for elimination. What can't be excreted will therefore remain inside the body and begin to accumulate in the cellular terrain.

### What about Toxic Substances?

Contrary to toxins, toxic substances should never be found in the body. These are substances that are totally foreign to normal body functions and are harmful to the organism; hence their description as toxic. All of the chemical poisons produced by pollution of the air, water, and soil (lead, cadmium, mercury, and so forth) are considered toxic substances.

An additional significant quantity of harmful foreign substances enters the body via common food additives, as well as the majority of pesticides, herbicides, and fungicides that are regularly used in industrial agriculture to treat food and animal products. Of the reported four thousand different compounds found in tobacco smoke, such as benzene, uranium, and formaldehyde, the American Cancer Society reports that at least seventy are known to cause cancer, and many others cause additional health problems. Certain medications and vaccines also contain toxic substances.

All of these toxic substances are difficult to eliminate, because the body is not designed to receive or discard them. Thanks to its detoxifying abilities, the liver is the organ best equipped to neutralize and eliminate them.

## Classification of Toxins and Toxic Substances by Entry Point

Toxins and toxic substances primarily enter the body by three distinct paths.

### Digestive Tract: Food and Beverage

- Excessive consumption of sugar, fats, protein, salt, and so on
- Food additives: colorings, preservatives, anti-rancidity products, and so on
- Pesticides, herbicides, and fungicides used in cultivation and production
- Medications, growth promoters, and antibiotics used in producing animal products
- Drugs and medications
- Polluted water and crops

## Respiratory Tract

+ Polluted air (industrial emissions, automobile emissions, and so forth)
+ Air that contains excessive particulate matter
+ Tobacco smoke

## Skin

+ Synthetic and non-organic cosmetics, talcum and other powders, creams, hair dye, shampoo, deodorant, hair conditioner, soap, and other personal care products

---

### ? Did You Know?

Overeating leads not only to becoming overweight but also to an overload of toxins. However, it's possible to suffer from a disproportionate quantity of toxins in your body and still not gain weight.

---

## THE EMUNCTORY ORGANS: EXIT DOORS FOR TOXINS

To maintain the purity of the physiological cellular terrain, the body has at its disposal five organs that filter toxins out of the bloodstream and expel them from the body. These organs are the liver, intestines, kidneys, skin (with its sudoriferous and sebaceous glands), and lungs.

These eliminatory organs are technically known as the *emunctory* organs, and they serve as exit doors for toxins in the body.

When these organs are working normally and the production and intake of toxins is not too high, the terrain

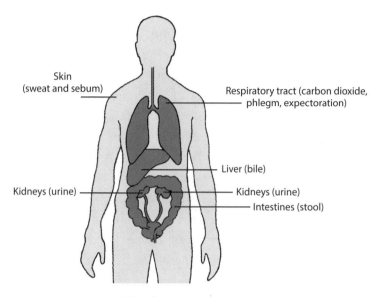

*The five emunctory organs*

remains clean. Cells can function properly because the excretory organs are eliminating the toxins at the same rate at which they are appearing.

On the other hand, when the quantities of toxins are too great, the eliminatory capacities of the organs are quickly exceeded and the terrain starts to gradually collect larger and larger amounts of toxins. If, in addition, the excretory organs are sluggish or deficient, the rate of increase of toxins will climb even higher and illness will result.

## DRAINING TOXINS

If a disease is due to accumulated toxins in the body, it is only logical that the ideal therapy would seek out and eliminate these toxins from the physical organism. This intentional elimination of toxins is performed by draining or purging, more commonly known today as detox.*

A purging consists of stimulating the function of the body's various excretory systems in order to accelerate the rate at which toxins are filtered out of the bloodstream and then eliminated from the body.

This stimulation of the emunctory organs can be performed by various means, called drainers—foods, medicinal herbs, massage, hydrotherapy—that have the ability to intensify the eliminatory capacities of an emunctory organ.

The emunctory organs are the essential means for draining or purging the body of harmful substances. In treatments that focus on intensifying the purging of the body, all efforts are concentrated on these organs. When eliminations have been insufficient, the target of the treatment is to restore a normal rate of elimination, or, even better, to temporarily accelerate it to compensate for the delay.

The distinguishing feature of a draining treatment is an increasing elimination of wastes by the emunctory organs. This increase in elimination should be readily apparent:

- Matter evacuated by the intestines will be more abundant or evacuations will occur more regularly.
- Urine will take on a darker color as it becomes charged with wastes and increases in volume.

---

*For more details about detoxing, see my book *Optimal Detox: How to Cleanse Your Body of Colloidal and Crystalline Toxins* (Healing Arts Press, 2011). For details about the benefits of a detox protocol that uses just one type of food, please see *The Detox Mono Diet: The Miracle Grape Cure and Other Cleansing Diets* (Healing Arts Press, 2006).

- The skin will perspire more profusely.
- The respiratory tract will discharge colloidal wastes that have been congesting it.

There will be a corresponding reduction of toxin levels in the tissues. Little by little, the cellular terrain will become clean again, and as a result, the symptoms of the disease will abate and gradually disappear. The body's organs will again be able to function properly because they will no longer be congested with toxins.

The possibilities for healing are obviously dependent on how much damage has already been inflicted on the organs by these wastes, as well as their natural ability to regenerate.

## THE ROLE OF THE LIVER

The liver is only one of the five excretory organs in the body. The liver is not more important than the other four for healthy overall body function, but it does, as we shall see, hold a very distinctive position.

Just like the other emunctory organs, the liver eliminates a large number of toxins. However, in addition to elimination it also neutralizes toxins. The other four excretory organs do not have this capability, or certainly not to the same extent. If they are able to neutralize toxins at all, it is to a much lesser degree.

---

### ⚠ Caution!

Although the liver's mission is to eliminate toxins and toxic substances, it can itself be overloaded by them.

---

For this reason, if any particular excretory organ needs to be in top working condition, it is the liver. Likewise, when it is necessary for a patient to stimulate an excretory organ due to poor bodily function, most often the most appropriate organ will be the liver. However, the liver absorbs so much abuse in its processing of both toxins and toxic substances that it can also be overwhelmed by them. If this is the case and their presence in large quantity is compromising proper liver function, detoxifying the liver takes priority in order to avoid risking the health of the rest of the body.

### Summary

- Disease is caused by an accumulation of toxins.
- The liver is one of the key organs for eliminating these harmful substances.
- The liver is capable of neutralizing both toxins and toxic substances.

# 2

# ANATOMY OF THE LIVER

*The liver is the paramount organ of our metabolism.*
SANDRA CABOT, M.D., MEDICAL DIRECTOR OF THE
AUSTRALIAN WOMEN'S HEALTH ADVISORY SERVICE

In order to take proper care of your liver, you need to understand it well. What does it look like? Where is it located in the body, and what is its relationship with the other organs of the body?

## THE LIVER REVEALED

The liver sits beneath the diaphragm, the dome-shaped muscle that serves as a partition separating the lungs and heart on one side and the abdominal organs—kidneys, intestines, and liver—on the other. The liver is located above a portion of the small intestine and beneath the right lung, where it is almost entirely protected from external shock by the ribs. Because of this, only a very small portion of the liver can be palpated by sliding the fingers beneath the rib cage.

The liver is the largest internal organ of the human body.

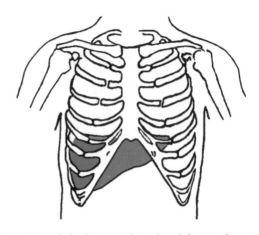

*Location of the liver within the abdominal cavity*

Reddish brown in color, with a smooth surface and solid consistency, it measures an average of 11 inches from left to right, 6 inches from front to back, and 4 inches from top to bottom. Compared to the kidneys, each of which is comparable in size to an average human fist, the mass of the liver is up to three times greater. Its healthy weight averages 5.5 pounds when engorged with blood within a living body and 3.3 pounds inside a cadaver. As we age, the liver decreases in volume by up to 40 percent, with a blood volume decrease from ages forty to sixty-five of 35 percent.

## THE LIVER AND THE CIRCULATORY SYSTEM

The liver is connected to the circulatory system by three vessels: the portal vein, the hepatic artery, and the hepatic vein. Two of these vessels enter the liver to supply it with blood, and the third delivers blood back out into general circulation.

## *The Portal Vein*

The capillaries located inside the intestinal walls combine to form the portal vein, which supplies 75 percent of blood flow to the liver. The role of the capillaries is to extract the nutrients from foods that are in the digestive tract. If the permeability of the intestinal mucous membranes is too high, because they have been injured by aggressive toxins, the capillaries will then also absorb whatever harmful substances are contained in the foods being digested.

Depending on circumstances, blood that flows through the portal vein will transport:

- Nutrients (amino acids, glucose, vitamins, and so forth)
- Food additives (preservatives, food coloring, and so on)
- Farming products used to treat food crops (insecticides, pesticides, herbicides, and so on)
- Pollutants (heavy metals, among other things)
- Toxic substances produced from food that ferments and putrefies inside the intestines
- Pharmaceutical medications and drugs

Because the majority of substances entering the body via the digestive tract get transported to the liver by the portal vein, this organ is the first defensive rampart of the body to

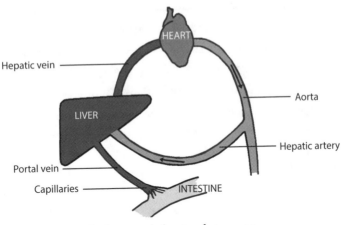

*The liver and the circulatory system*

face the molecules coming from outside, and the first organ that can act against them as a selective filter.

### The Hepatic Artery

The aorta, the largest artery in the human body, distributes oxygen-rich blood from the heart via several branches. One of these branches is the hepatic artery, which brings oxygenated blood to the liver so it is able to function properly.

---

 **Good to Know**

Blood flow into the liver can be broken down as follows:

- 25 percent via the hepatic artery
- 75 percent via the portal vein

---

### The Hepatic Vein

After entering the liver, the portal vein and the hepatic artery branch off into very thin blood vessels known as the sinusoidal capillaries, or simply sinusoids, where the oxygen-rich blood from the hepatic artery mixes with the nutrient-rich blood from the portal vein. These vessels bring the blood into close contact with the hepatic cells, or hepatocytes, which comprise the bulk of the liver mass and perform most of its functions, taking nutritive substances from the bloodstream and ridding the blood of undesirable substances. The sinusoidal capillaries then recombine to form the hepatic vein that takes deoxygenated blood by way of the inferior vena cava back into the heart, and from there back into general circulation.

The blood that circulates in the hepatic vein transports:

- Nutrients the body can utilize in their existing state
- Nutrients the liver has transformed so that they can be utilized
- Very few toxins, as the role of the liver is to filter them out of the bloodstream and eliminate them in the bile

Every minute, 1½ quarts of blood are processed through the liver, equal to one quarter of the body's entire blood output. Clearly this is a very important gland.

## THE LIVER AND
## THE DIGESTIVE SYSTEM

The liver is connected to the digestive system by means of the bile ducts. The liver cells extract toxins from the blood that is circulating through the sinusoidal capillaries and then expel them in the form of bile into thin tubes or channels known as the bile *canaliculi*.

The bile canaliculi combine to form the left and right hepatic ducts, each of which drains its corresponding side of the liver. These two channels converge to form the common hepatic duct that emerges from the liver and extends as the bile duct. This duct terminates in the duodenum, which is located directly at the exit of the stomach. The duodenum is, in fact, the beginning of the small intestine. The end of the bile duct at the entrance to the duodenum is equipped with a muscular valve—the sphincter of Oddi—that regulates the passage of bile. Where the hepatic duct meets the bile duct, we have the cystic duct. It carries a portion of the bile to the gallbladder, which is a storage pocket for the bile needed for digestion of fats that will come through the pipeline after your next meal.

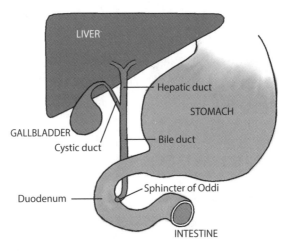

*The bile ducts*

The bile that makes its way into the intestine therefore contains:

- Digestive juices necessary for the digestion of fats
- Toxins that have been neutralized by the liver and are to be eliminated from the body via the stool

## THE LIVER AND THE INTESTINES

A close relationship exists between the liver and the intestines, by means of the portal vein. Any malfunction or defect in one of these two organs will have repercussions in the other.

Everything that is absorbed from the intestinal contents, whether nutrients or toxins, is transported directly into the liver by means of the portal vein. As it happens, the quantity of toxins transported into the liver greatly depends on the state of the intestines.

---

### ? Did You Know?

More than any other organ, the liver has the ability to rebuild a portion—even a very large portion—of its tissues so long as they have not been totally destroyed or surgically removed. In the best-case scenario, the removal of 75 percent of hepatic mass will not prevent the liver from rebuilding its missing tissue. In a matter of four months the liver will recover its usual weight and shape.

---

When the intestinal transit is normal (one stool per day) and when the intestinal mucous membranes that filter wastes are in good shape, this quantity is minimal. The situation changes when the intestines stop functioning properly. A slowing of the intestinal transit will increase the time during which toxins remain in contact with the mucous membranes of the intestinal walls, thus allowing them more time to be absorbed. This is how too many toxins are able to enter the bloodstream and make their way into the liver. The quantities become even higher if the intestines are sluggish, meaning that the individual has severe constipation.

Prolonged contact of toxins with the intestinal mucous

membranes also increases the time during which toxins and toxic substances can damage the intestinal walls. The prolonged contact causes microlesions that function as open portals allowing undesirable substances to enter the bloodstream and thereby be transported to the liver.

This increased presence of toxins will exhaust the liver, which will weaken it and make it impossible for it to produce sufficient bile. The decrease in bile will slow the intestinal transit still further. However, the slower the intestinal transit becomes, the more toxins are absorbed by the bloodstream and carried into the liver. This establishes a veritable vicious cycle.

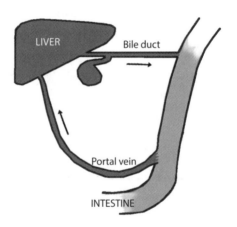

*The liver and the intestines*

### Summary

- The liver is located on the right side of the rib cage.
- It is one of the largest and most important organs of the body.
- It is the first organ to receive the substances absorbed by the intestines.

# 3

# ROLE AND FUNCTION
# OF THE LIVER

*The liver is a miraculous factory.*

PIERRE-VALENTIN MARCHESSEAU,
FOUNDER OF THE FIRST FREE UNIVERSITY
OF NATUROPATHY IN PARIS IN 1935

The multiple functions of the liver can be broken down into two general functions:

♦ To produce the numerous molecules necessary for the body (nutrition)
♦ To rid the body of detrimental toxins and pathogens (elimination and defense)

## ? Did You Know?

The many activities of the liver produce heat and raise its temperature. The liver is generally 102.2° to 105.8°F—that is, hotter than the rest of the body. If we eat a lot, this increases the temperature of the liver even more, which is communicated to the rest of the body. This explains why we feel warm when we are eating a large meal.

## AN ORGAN WITH MULTIPLE FUNCTIONS

The liver fulfills more than five hundred functions. No other organ performs as many different tasks. Amazingly, the liver performs all of these tasks simultaneously.

---

### ? Did You Know?

The importance of the liver for life is revealed by its etymology. In English, the word *liver* is quite close to the word *live*. The same is true in German, where liver (*leber*) and life (*leben*) are quite close.

---

### *Storage of Glucose and Regulation of Glycemia*

The energetic fuel that the cells use is the sugar known as glucose. To compensate for the inconsistent supply of glucose from food due to time intervals between meals, the liver transforms glucose into glycogen. The liver then stores this substance in its tissues as a reserve, to be supplied to the blood as needed. Every time the blood sugar (glycemia) drops, the liver converts this glycogen back into glucose, which it then discharges into the bloodstream in order to maintain the optimal glycemia level for proper functioning of the body. If we did not have a liver, we would be constantly running out of energy.

If the foods we eat do not bring in enough carbohydrates to be transformed into glycogen, the liver will manufacture them from fats or proteins. In the contrary situation, when we are ingesting too many carbohydrates and the liver's glycogen reserves are full, excess sugars are stored in the liver in the form of fat. This fatty overload weakens the liver and hinders it from functioning properly.

*Storage of Nutrients and Regulation of Levels*
In addition to glucose, the liver stores all kinds of other nutrients:

◆ Vitamins A and D
◆ Various B vitamins, such as vitamin $B_{12}$, a deficiency of which can cause pernicious anemia
◆ Iron, copper, and so on

When the blood level of any of these nutrients falls, the liver releases more into the bloodstream to bring it back to normal. If the liver lacks these nutrients, deficiency illnesses appear.

*Production of Proteins*
The amino acids entering the liver by the portal vein are transformed there into different proteins that are useful to the body. These include:

◆ *Albumin:* This is the form taken by the proteins of the blood and muscles.
◆ *Prothrombin and fibrinogen:* In the event of a wound, these proteins cause blood to coagulate and form into clots that seal the cut vessels. This is how the body prevents total blood loss.
◆ *Carrier proteins:* These are the substances used by the blood for transport. Lipids, hormones, medications, and so forth do not independently circulate in the blood but are transported by a special support with a protein base. For example, the lipoproteins carry fats (including cholesterol, which otherwise would adhere to the blood vessel walls), glycoproteins ensure the transport of sexual hormones in the blood, and so forth.
◆ *Proinflammatory proteins:* These proteins (cytokines)

trigger the defensive reaction of inflammation, which allows the cells to destroy any injurious agent that threatens their physical integrity.

The liver does not store proteins. It transforms excess proteins into urea, which is then sent on to the kidneys. This transformation is hard work for the liver.

*Prolonged protein overloads will eventually exhaust the liver and cause it to deteriorate.*

### *Metabolism of Fats*

The liver synthesizes lipids that are helpful to the body, such as phospholipids. It can either send these substances directly into the bloodstream or store them in its reserves to cover future needs. When the liver has to store too many fats, which is the case when we eat too much food with lipids, it becomes congested with fats, a condition that can lead to the fatty degeneration of the liver.

Common factors that can lead to a fatty liver include:

- Obesity
- High levels of fat in the blood
- Diabetes
- Genetic propensity
- Rapid weight loss
- Side effect of some medications

---

### ? **Did You Know?**

*Gourmet treat!?* The foie gras eaten by gourmets and gastronomes is made from liver that has deliberately been congested with fats when geese are force-fed. This culinary indulgence is actually made from a diseased liver.

---

### *Purification or Detoxification of Blood*

The bloodstream carries numerous toxins, which are the metabolic residues and wastes produced by the body performing its functions. The liver is one of the organs responsible for filtering these substances out of the blood so they can be eliminated from the body. The liver performs this task by diluting them in bile, which allows them to exit the body in the stool.

### *Defense against Harmful Agents and Their Destruction*

Thanks to specialized cells known as Kupffer cells (see page 35), the liver destroys everything that threatens the physical integrity of the body—in other words, germs, toxic substances, carcinogens, carcinogenic cells, and so on. The liver is the only organ in the body capable of doing this.

## HOW THE LIVER WORKS

The defensive abilities of the liver are highly effective as long as the liver is functioning well.

To understand the liver's importance for health and learn how to support its efforts, it helps to have a more detailed description of the various ways it functions.

### *Blood Purification*

Purification of the blood—the elimination of the toxins and toxic substances it contains—is critical because the accumulation of undesirable and injurious substances in the body's cellular terrain is the source of the vast majority of our diseases.

These toxins and toxic substances can wreak havoc when allowed to persist. They:

- Thicken the blood and clog blood vessels (cardiovascular diseases)
- Attack the joints (arthritis, rheumatism)
- Clog the respiratory tract (bronchitis, colds, asthma, and so on)
- Saturate the skin (pimples, eczema, and other skin disorders)
- Form clusters in the organs (such as kidney or bile stones)
- Form deposits on the tissues (cellulitis, obesity)
- Alter cellular function (cancer)

The filtration and elimination of toxins is performed by hepatocyte cells, the basic building blocks of the liver. They represent 80 percent of the cells in the liver, with the remainder being the Kupffer cells mentioned earlier with regard to their defense against, and destruction of, any pathogens or other harmful agents that threaten the body's physical integrity.

### Hepatocytes

The liver is crisscrossed by countless sinusoidal capillaries that branch off from the portal vein. The entire length of these capillaries is surrounded by hepatocytes, which effectively form a layer that envelops every sinusoidal capillary. The walls of these capillaries are pierced with tiny "windows" that permit toxins to leave

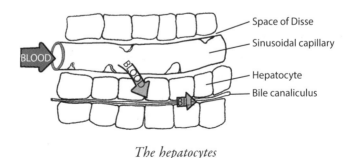

*The hepatocytes*

the bloodstream and encounter the hepatocytes. This meeting takes place in the perisinusoidal space between the hepatocytes and the walls of the capillaries. Known as the space of Disse, it is filled with blood. Microvillae of hepatocytes extend into this space, absorbing components of the sinusoids.

Toxins and toxic substances that enter into contact with the hepatocytes have a variety of origins. They can be:

### TOXINS

+ Protein wastes (urea)
+ Wastes from fats (cholesterol, saturated fatty acids)
+ Poisons produced by intestinal fermentation and putrefaction (indoles, scatoles, and so on)
+ Carbohydrate waste products (acids, flocculants, and so on)
+ Mineral waste (sodium, chlorine, potassium, and so forth)
+ Hormone waste
+ Cell cadavers (for example, of red blood cells)

### TOXIC SUBSTANCES

+ Alcohol
+ Medications
+ Antibiotics
+ Heavy metals from pollution
+ Coloring agents and other food additives
+ Pesticides
+ Tobacco

The purification of the blood by the hepatocytes is an active task. Contrary to the kidneys, where blood filtering takes place in a more passive manner thanks to the pressure of the blood crossing through the renal filter, the liver works actively to capture toxins and toxic substances and to transform their characteristics. In other words, it actively seeks to neutralize and deactivate them. This causes them to become harmless so they can be eliminated without posing a threat to other parts of the body.

---

### ⚠ Caution!

Alcohol is not a food but a poison the body seeks to expunge by neutralizing it. The liver plays a supremely important role in this case as it neutralizes 95 percent of the alcohol ingested by the body. Even when just drinking "a little," you are making a lot of work for your liver. Over a year's time, daily consumption of 1¼ cups of wine with 12 percent alcohol content adds up to 15 quarts of pure alcohol.

---

This task of transformation and neutralization takes place in two stages.

### Phase 1

This phase consists of transforming the harmful substances using a variety of procedures:

- Oxidation: the substance combines with oxygen.
- Reduction: oxygen is removed from the substance.
- Hydrolysis: the chemical substance is broken down by dilution with water.

These chemical transformations take place thanks to large numbers of enzymes in the hepatocytes. One of the most important of these enzymes is cytochrome oxidase P450.

Phase 2

This phase involves the neutralization and deactivation of harmful substances. The process used here is that of conjugation, meaning the toxin or toxic substance is combined with another molecule, one that possesses the necessary characteristics for neutralizing harmful effects. Glucuronic acid is the most common molecule used to achieve conjugation.

Toxins and toxic substances that have been neutralized in this way will then be released by the hepatocytes along with other substances to form bile.

### *The Defense of the Body and the Destruction of Assailants*

In addition to toxins produced by the body's normal functioning—which is top priority for the hepatocytes—the liver has other specialized cells at its disposal to defend itself against both external and internal assaults that threaten the physical integrity of the body. These are the previously mentioned Kupffer cells.

---

### 🖐 **Good to Know**

The cellular division of the liver:

- Hepatocytes: 80 percent
- Kupffer cells: 20 percent

---

Kupffer Cells

Kupffer cells are not fixed in place the way hepatocytes are but are mobile. Their location in the sinusoidal capillaries puts them in direct contact with all the blood that enters the liver, as they are effectively immersed in that blood.

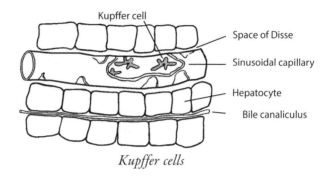

*Kupffer cells*

Kupffer cells are macrophages, meaning they are large in size (*macro*) and have the ability to swallow and digest (*phage*), by which process they can destroy all threats that have not already been neutralized and eliminated by hepatocytes. These injurious substances are primarily:

- Dead or diseased cells
- Cancerous cells (metastatic cells transported by the bloodstream)
- Poorly digested proteins coming from the intestines
- Bacteria
- Viruses
- Parasites (amoebas, malaria plasmodia, and so forth)
- Yeast (*Candida albicans*)
- Medications
- Undesirable chemical substances (herbicides, pesticides, antioxidants, preservatives, and so on)
- Synthetic substances
- Carcinogenic substances
- Drugs
- Heavy metals
- Toxic substances caused by pollution

**Good to Know**

*Watch out! Alien proteins!* While all proteins are made up of the same basic amino acids, every living human being has a uniquely personal sequence of amino acids according to individual genetic code. The immune system knows how to tell the difference between personal proteins and those that are foreign, and it destroys proteins it detects as alien: germs, animal secretions (venom), plant tissues (poisons), and so on that are dangerous for the body. When we eat proteins (such as those in fish or meat), the body recognizes the animal flesh as "other protein" not a personal protein and so breaks it down.

 **Good to Know**

"The number of medications now recognized as hepatotoxic [damaging to liver cells] has grown considerably. This is due, in part, to the introduction of new molecules, but also to the late recognition of the hepatotoxicity of older medicines. Currently more than six hundred medications are suspected of hepatotoxicity."

DOMINIQUE PESSAYRE, M.D., HEPATIC PATHOLOGY SPECIALIST

Kupffer cells use enzymes to help them "digest" pathogens. The aggressor is killed if it is a living entity (germ or cell) or destroyed if it is a toxic molecule or substance. In either case, the pathogen is broken down into smaller, inoffensive particles. In this way Kupffer cells rid the blood of all aggressive elements.

Kupffer cells have the capacity to perform enormous tasks, but like all workers, they require time to digest and recuperate. When they are overworked, which is the case when multiple forms of intoxication are involved (medications, tobacco, drugs, alcohol, and so forth), they are less effective. They absorb fewer of the invasive entities and do not digest them properly. The toxic substances evade them and worm their way more deeply into the body.

### Kupffer Cells and the Immune System

There are numerous kinds of macrophages in the body, found in bone marrow, brain, spleen, and so on. Wherever they reside, they belong to the immune system, whose job is to protect the self (the body) from the non-self (germs, cancerous cells, toxic substances, and so on). The Kupffer cells do not work any differently from other macrophages located in the various organs of the body, but they do constitute 80 to 90 percent of the tissue-resident macrophages in the whole body. Their reputation as powerful defenders is due to their extremely high number. Remember, they represent a significant percentage of the cells of the liver, an organ already known for its large size! Kupffer cells are the "secret weapon" of the liver that make it a powerful defender of the body.

---

### ? Did You Know?

Bacteria, viruses, and yeast make up the huge family of microbes that are hazardous to humans, but the liver is capable of destroying them. The immune system is therefore not the only one to kill microbes; the liver does it too.

---

The importance of the liver also arises from the fact that it is the first barrier of macrophages encountered by food substances, medications, drugs, pollutants, and so on arriving from the intestines. As long as the liver remains healthy, these harmful substances cannot invade the body to collect in the terrain but are destroyed before they manage to get any farther. However, when the liver has been overworked and weakened, they enter the bloodstream and then the tissues. The other macrophages of the immune system then go into action to prevent the degradation of the cellular terrain and the onset of disease. Whether or not their efforts are rewarded with success depends on the quantity of toxins that reach them.

### The Production of Bile for the Digestion of Fats

The bile secreted by the hepatocytes is collected by little tubes known as the bile *canaliculi*. These small tubes combine to form larger ones that in turn form the hepatic channel, through which the bile is conducted to the gallbladder and intestines.

The role played by bile is twofold:

- It supports the elimination of toxins and toxic substances, which requires a continuous secretion as well as constant elimination toward the intestine.
- It aids the digestion and absorption of lipids (fats) in the small intestine, something that requires a periodic excretion (at every meal).

The realization of these two opposing imperatives is possible thanks to the gallbladder. The bile being continually released by the liver can flow directly and without interruption toward the intestine by passing through the hepatic and bile ducts, which serve to eliminate toxins. The gallbladder, meanwhile, in its capacity as a reservoir can store a certain quantity of bile, which guarantees its periodic availability for the digestion of meals.

### Bile

The liver releases around 1 quart of bile every day. This is a limpid, viscous fluid that has an alkaline pH (7.6 to 8.6). Bile is yellow in color and has a bitter flavor. (This explains why some-one who is bitter and angry may be described as "full of bile.")

The bile stored in the gallbladder is more concentrated than that which flows directly into the intestine. The color of this bile is also different; it is olive green.

The components of bile are:

- Water
- Bile salts
- Bilirubin
- Cholesterol
- Lecithin
- Various minerals

Bile salts have an emulsifying action, meaning they divide fats into droplets, which allows the pancreatic lipase to digest them completely. This preparation of the fats by the bile salts encourages the absorption of liposoluble (fat-soluble) vitamins—vitamins A, D, E, K, and omega-3 and omega-6.

When there are liver deficiencies, there is poor absorption of fat-soluble vitamins and the appearance of deficiency diseases with a decline in overall health.

A lack of bile salts in the gallbladder will result in inferior emulsification of the cholesterol contained in bile, and hence the risk of cholesterol solidifying, which could result in gallstones.

Bilirubin is a bile pigment or substance resulting from the breakdown of blood hemoglobin. It plays no digestive role but is a waste that should be eliminated. Its brownish-yellow tinge gives stool their characteristic coloration. In someone suffer-ing from hepatitis, the bile ducts are congested so severely that bilirubin can no longer flow into the intestines, the stools become colorless, and bilirubin travels into the bloodstream, giving a yellow tinge to the skin and the whites of the eyes and a mahogany color to urine.

Cholesterol is fundamentally a beneficial substance but can become harmful when present in overly large quantities in the body. This is why the liver expels cholesterol into the bile when necessary. Because it is not soluble in water, cholesterol cannot remain suspended in this liquid. It is able to maintain a state of suspension in the bile thanks to the actions of bile salts and lecithin. If these latter substances are missing, the cholesterol particles will precipitate (separate out and clump) and form stones in the gallbladder.

Lecithin is an emulsifier, meaning it helps to make fats soluble. Their digestion is facilitated, which also lessens the risk that they will form deposits in the blood vessels. In fact, lecithin lowers high blood cholesterol.

---

### ✚ Tips and Tricks

Lecithin is sold in the form of pleasant-tasting granulated pellets and capsules. The recommended daily dose of the granulated form is 2 to 4 tablespoons a day, which can be eaten plain. Granulated lecithin can also be mixed with food or stirred into a drink.

The content of the capsules varies from one manufacturer to another, so it's best to follow dosage instructions provided by the manufacturer.

---

### The Functioning of the Gallbladder

Bile is stored in the gallbladder for digestive purposes. When you eat a meal, the food passes through your stomach and reaches the duodenum, where receptors detect the arrival of fats. These receptors then send neural and hormonal signals alerting the gallbladder to provide the bile it has set aside for this purpose. The different processes in play are comprised of three steps:

1. Food triggers the emptying of the gallbladder. When the gallbladder is informed of the arrival of fats in the duodenum, it contracts three or four times to evacuate the bile it is holding. These contractions are vigorous, as they are also intended to move the bile first through the cystic duct and then the bile duct.

2. Postprandial period: The gallbladder is empty once it has sent its contents to the intestines to help digest a meal. It remains empty for some period of time while the bile the liver is continuing to produce is routed not toward the gallbladder but directly to the intestines to additionally facilitate digestion.

3. Interprandial period: Between meals, the now-empty gallbladder must be refilled so that it's ready to help with digestion of the next meal. Because the intestine is "fasting" at this time, it no longer needs any bile to help digest food from the previous meal, which has now worked its way much farther down the digestive tube.

---

## ? Did You Know?

When the gallbladder has collected too many bile stones and is no longer capable of storing and expelling bile, surgery is required to remove the gallbladder. Digestion will now take place with only the bile that is continuously released by the liver. Because this means there is less bile available for digestion, it's a good idea to eat smaller meals and consume less fat.

---

The gallbladder refills with bile thanks to the closing of the sphincter of Oddi, a valve that controls the flow of bile and pancreatic juice. The bile that continues to be produced by the liver can no longer enter the intestines, as its forward movement is blocked by the sphincter of Oddi. It flows back into the bile and cystic ducts and starts collecting in the gall-bladder. In order to reduce the volume of bile that needs to be stored, the gallbladder concentrates it by removing a portion of its water. A concentrated and consequently highly active bile is therefore prepared for the arrival of the next meal.

---

### Summary

- The liver possesses more than five hundred functions. Among these, it regulates the rate of sugar and vitamins in the bloodstream, produces proteins and lipids, removes toxins from the bloodstream, and destroys germs and toxic substances.

- The liver is comprised of 80 percent hepatocytes and 20 percent Kupffer cells. The hepatocytes extract toxins from the bloodstream. Kupffer cells neutralize toxic substances.

- Bile is both a digestive juice and a support for the elimination of wastes. The bile of the gallbladder is released during meals. Its higher concentration encourages better digestion of fats.

---

# 4

# DISEASES OF THE LIVER

The liver, like any other organ, can fall ill. The diseases that afflict it are primarily due to the overwork imposed upon it by overeating, chemical pollution of food, alcohol, overmedication, and stimulants.

## LIVER DEFICIENCY

In the event of hepatic deficiency, the liver, although not truly ill, is not functioning as well as it should. It is weak and lethargic, and thus often described as "sluggish liver." When the liver is in this state, it is congested, meaning that blood and toxins are stagnating within it. This congestion slows the production and release of bile.

Sluggish liver can be more or less pronounced, depending on the individual. The health problems this can cause are legion and can affect all parts of the body, as any kind of hepatic deficiency will inevitably lead to an overload of toxins in the terrain, which is the starting point for disease. However, the first troubles to appear will be in the digestive sphere. They are also the most visible and easiest to detect.

A person suffering from hepatic deficiency will not necessarily be affected by all of these problems, but usually several are relevant:

- Difficulty digesting fats (eggs, cream, high-fat meals, and so on)
- Digestive troubles in general
- Bouts of nausea
- Swelling and feeling heavy around the belly
- Gas or bloating
- Pasty tongue
- Bad breath
- Loss of appetite
- Fatigue and lack of enthusiasm
- Yellowish tinge to the skin and eyes
- Constipation
- Gallstones
- Itching on the skin
- Hemorrhoids

Minor hepatic deficiency is not serious but will impair the quality of life. Someone suffering from this problem will constantly be forced to deal with digestive disorders and be continually tired and lacking in vitality and enthusiasm. It is only when the deficiency becomes pronounced that the cellular terrain begins to break down and other organs start to be affected.

## BILE STONES

The liver is constantly producing bile. While one portion of this bile is carried directly into the intestines by the bile duct, the rest—a little less than half—is set aside in reserve in the gallbladder to be used for digestion of the next meal. In order to reduce the volume of bile to be stored, the mucous membranes of the gallbladder reabsorb some of the water it contains, bringing the bile's rate of water content from 97.5 percent down to 87 percent. When this happens, the concentration of solid substances in the bile obviously increases. For example, the amount of bile salts goes from 1 percent to 6 percent.

## BILE COMPOSITION

|  | Liver Bile | Gallbladder Bile |
|---|---|---|
| **Water** | 97.5% | 87% |
| **Bile salts** | 1.1% | 6% |
| **Cholesterol** | 0.1% | 0.3–0.9% |
| **Bilirubin** | 0.04% | 0.3% |
| **Lecithin** | 0.04% | 0.3% |

The composition of bile in the liver is, therefore, different from that of the bile stored in the gallbladder, which is four to five times more concentrated, stringy, and viscous. The higher viscosity of gallbladder bile is a benefit for digestion, as it contains a higher content of digestive juices. However, it does expose the individual to one danger: the saturation point is close, and at that point the substances being held in suspension will precipitate and form bile stones.

*The principal cause for the formation of bile stones is overeating.*

Meals that are too rich and too frequent will wear out the gallbladder. Its walls will lose their tone. The bile this organ contains will then be ejected imperfectly into the intestine during the course of a meal. One portion will remain in the gallbladder, and therefore at risk of becoming even more highly concentrated. In this way, little by little, the gallbladder will retain a stock of stagnant bile. The cholesterol and mineral salts it contains will inevitably precipitate. This is the phenomenon that occurs when a substance that is part of a fluid solution becomes solid and forms a deposit. The salts and cholesterol that had been dissolved and suspended in the bile will fall to the bottom of the organ. Initially these substances remain isolated, but eventually they begin to clump. This state is typically described as biliary sludge, which is thick bile that can lead to the formation of tiny crystals and finally bile stones that can grow to several centimeters in size.

Bile stones are not innately dangerous, but by collecting in the gallbladder they hinder its proper functioning.

When the bile required for digestion is no longer coming into the small intestine in its regular quantities, digestive problems occur. The thick bile that is stagnating in the gallbladder irritates those mucous membranes, which leads to inflammation and then sclerosis. The environment this creates is especially susceptible to infection. The greatest danger, though, is when a bile stone exits the gallbladder. If it is larger than any portion of the bile duct or cystic duct (which connects the gallbladder and common bile duct), it can become stuck in one of these two tubes. This will result in severe pain (liver colic) and a local liver infection (hepatitis or jaundice).

---

### 🖐 Good to Know

The formation of bile stones begins with the presence of sludge or thick bile that precipitates and forms crystals. When these microparticles clump together, they form bile stones.

---

## VARIETIES OF HEPATITIS

Hepatitis attacks are liver inflammations.* They are considered acute disorders, characterized by their intensity and generally short duration.

During a hepatitis attack, the liver tissues become swollen. They crush the bile ducts, which blocks the flow of bile and prevents it from passing into the intestines. Some of this blocked bile stagnates in the liver, hindering its detoxifying functions. The rest makes its way into the bloodstream. Because it contains a number of toxins, once it is freely circulating in the blood it can ultimately poison the body.

Hepatitis symptoms are very easy to see. They are primarily connected to bilirubin, the yellow pigment in bile, which in the course of this disease is dispersed throughout the body. They include:

- Yellow coloration, or jaundice (from the French word for yellow: *jaune*) of the skin and the whites of the eyes
- Darker urine (the typical yellow color of urine is caused by the presence of bilirubin)
- Discolored stools (as they are not receiving the bilirubin they normally obtain from the bile sent to the intestines)

Someone with hepatitis also suffers from:

- Fatigue
- Loss of appetite
- Episodic fevers
- Itching

---

*For a more comprehensive discussion of inflammation, please see my book *Natural Remedies for Inflammation* (Healing Arts Press, 2014).

Hepatitis can have a variety of causes, including anything that irritates the bile ducts and triggers inflammation that obstructs and clogs them. Its various forms are distinguished as follows:

- *Viral hepatitis:* The attack is due to a virus.
- *Toxic hepatitis:* The attack is due to poison or medication.
- *Mechanical hepatitis:* A bile stone blocks the bile ducts.
- *Hemolytic hepatitis:* There is an excess of hemoglobin to be broken down (often caused by incompatibility of blood types between mother and child, or as the result of a blood transfusion).

---

### ? Did You Know?

The liver can be affected by different types of viral hepatitis. There are three predominant types, each of which is identified with a letter.

- Hepatitis A is transmitted via drinking water or food that has been washed with infected water (such as salad greens, raw vegetables, fruits, or shellfish). Hepatitis A is generally of short duration and heals without any complications.
- Hepatitis B is transmitted by blood, and consequently this infection can be passed on by unsterilized syringes and other contaminated instruments (needles). It can also be transmitted by sexual relations. It can generally be remedied without any major complications.
- Hepatitis C is also transmitted by blood. Hepatitis C is problematic because it can develop into a debilitating chronic condition.

---

## CIRRHOSIS

When the liver has suffered repeated and numerous attacks over a period of time, lesional disorders take root. Cirrhosis in any form is a serious and chronic disease, as the liver's mass is being assaulted. The destruction of tissue causes first lesions, then scarring (fibrosis). Generally the liver's ability to regenerate is high, but in the chronic stage this regeneration cannot take place properly. It produces an excessive number of fibrous tissues that harden the liver and slow cellular exchange. The result is inevitably a disruption of liver function. The organ becomes increasingly incapable of properly performing its tasks of protection, detoxification, and bile production, as well as its many other functions.

---

### ⚠ Caution!

Cirrhosis is the culmination of a lifestyle that shows no respect for the liver. Seventy percent of all cirrhosis diseases are due to alcoholism.

---

The appearance of the liver changes completely. Instead of being smooth, firm, and a deep brown color, its surface becomes pitted. It becomes very hard to the touch and takes on a red color. The word *cirrhosis* draws its origin from this color; in Greek, *kirros* means "red."

## SEVERAL DISEASES CAUSED BY POOR LIVER FUNCTION

The repercussions of a shortfall in liver function can affect organs that are not even close to the liver. A superficial examination may give the impression that there is no connection between the liver and the ailing organs, but keeping in mind the role of the terrain and toxins in the origins of disease, the relationship becomes obvious.

## The Liver and the Mind

Various popular expressions in many languages reveal that human beings have often found a connection between mind and liver.

In French, someone who remains calm and is not easily disturbed is said to have "good liver." Someone who lacks courage is said to be "lily-livered" (colorless compared to the typical reddish brown). Someone who is overly excitable and prone to temper tantrums is said to "spill his bile," or vitriol. To urge someone to calm down, ancient Babylonians would say, "May your liver be smooth."

The term "bilious" has two contradictory definitions. Sometimes the word is used to describe a person who is anxious and worries about everything, and at other times it describes someone who is bad-tempered and impatient. The explanation for these two opposing moods is neither an overabundance nor a dearth of bile (to be bilious means you have too much bile), but according to anthroposophical doctor Victor Bott, M.D., it relates to biliary resorption in the intestines.

The way it works is that the bulk of the bile produced by the liver is expelled from the body through the stool, leaving a small portion behind to be absorbed by intestinal mucous membranes. According to Dr. Bott, when the resorption is too intense, we are irritable and quick to inflame. When it is too weak, we feel sluggish, apathetic, and peevish. In either case the result is the same: we feel out of sorts and generally unpleasant.

## *The Digestive Tract*

The first diseases that are engendered by deficiencies in liver function generally appear in the digestive tract, which makes sense given that the liver has a direct connection to this organ.

### Indigestion

On the digestive (and not eliminatory) level, the role played by the liver is twofold. In the first place, bile emulsifies fats, breaking them down into tiny particles that will next be attacked by the digestive juices of the pancreas and intestines. If this first stage is not achieved properly, fats not sufficiently transformed will cause bouts of nausea, a sense of heaviness, and the very real sensation that you have not digested your meal.

The second way the liver plays a part in digestion is by alkalizing the alimentary bolus, the mass of food from your last meal that is passing through the gastrointestinal tract. In order to digest proteins, the stomach secretes extremely acidic digestive juices. When the alimentary bolus first exits the stomach it has a pH of 2.5. However, the pancreatic and intestinal juices that are active in the intestines can be effective only in an alkaline environment—that is, with a pH above 7. The liver is responsible for changing the pH of the alimentary bolus to the level required by these digestive juices to function effectively. The bile it releases is highly alkaline, with a pH that ranges from 7.6 to 8.6. This alkalizes the alimentary bolus and in this way encourages the complete and effective digestion of fats. However, if an individual is suffering from liver deficiency, this alkalizing activity will not be sufficient. The fats will remain poorly digested and a variety of digestive disorders will manifest.*

---

*For a thorough description of how to maintain a healthy acid-alkaline balance, see my book *The Acid-Alkaline Diet for Optimum Health: Restore Your Health by Creating pH Balance in Your Diet* (Healing Arts Press, 2006).

### Constipation

The causes mentioned most often for constipation are a lack of roughage, lack of exercise, and insufficient liquid. But a frequently overlooked cause is liver deficiency. A sluggish liver will not release enough bile, and one of the properties of bile is to stimulate intestinal peristalsis, which moves digested food through the intestinal tract. So it is not only dietary fiber that triggers the contraction of the intestinal muscles but also bile. A sufficient secretion of bile consequently permits the stools to advance through the intestines even if there is a slight lack of roughage in the diet.

When there is a lack of bile, the intestines slow their activity. The partially digested matter sits stagnant and begins to accumulate, which makes the task of the peristaltic muscles more difficult. This is when constipation becomes an issue.

Bile also has the role of a lubricant, making the stool moist and slippery, which hugely facilitates progress through the intestines. It stops the stool from adhering to the mucous membranes of the intestinal walls, which are also made slippery by bile. This means that the stool can advance easily.

A lack of bile, on the other hand, makes stool sticky, which hampers its progress.

## Blood and the Circulatory System

Following the digestive system, the blood and circulatory system is most likely to be adversely affected by hepatic deficiency. Wastes that have been poorly neutralized and not completely eliminated by the liver collect in the bloodstream and form deposits on the vessel walls. Among the diseases this causes, we find the following.

### High Cholesterol

All the fats we consume go directly to the liver. The body uses only a portion of this quantity, and the remainder is transformed into cholesterol and triglycerides that the liver will expel into the bile. This product then passes into the intestines, from where, normally, it is evacuated with the stool, if there is sufficient roughage (whole grain husks, plant fibers of fruits and vegetables) to capture it. Fiber is essential for transporting cholesterol out of the body. It acts as a fine-mesh net that traps it. If there is insufficient fiber, the cholesterol will not be trapped and will be reabsorbed by the body. If you don't have enough fiber in your diet, up to 90 percent of cholesterol can be reabsorbed by the intestinal walls and taken back to the liver.

The surplus cholesterol that is returned this way to the liver will not be reprocessed and eliminated again by this organ but instead finds its way into general circulation. Because it is in excess quantities, it accumulates in the bloodstream (hypercholesterolemia) and begins forming deposits on the walls of the blood vessels. Thickening of the blood and the formation of fatty deposits are the basic causes of cardiovascular disease.

High blood cholesterol is reduced through both dietary adjustments and regular, intense stimulation of the liver, among other treatments such as exercise and relaxation.

---

### 🖐 Good to Know

Cholesterol is manufactured not only from a surplus of fats but also from an excess of sugar and protein.

---

### Cardiovascular Diseases

Cardiovascular diseases (thick blood or hyperviscosity, high blood pressure, heart attack, stroke, and so on) are many and varied in their expression, but they all fundamentally stem from the same cause: the accumulation of fatty substances in the bloodstream.

These substances thicken the blood, which slows its rate of circulation. When they are deposited on the walls of the blood vessels, they form fatty lumps (atheromas) in the arteries, reducing their diameter and impeding the passage of blood. When blood becomes too thick and stagnant, it coagulates. The clot this forms can clog a vessel in the heart (heart attack), in the brain (stroke), or elsewhere in the body (embolism).

These surplus fatty substances are, however, substances that the liver could have prevented from entering the bloodstream, had it not been overwhelmed by a diet high in "bad" fats and sugars.

Stimulating and detoxifying the liver, therefore, is an integral part of any treatment for cardiovascular disease.

---

### ? Did You Know?

Millions of people take blood thinners to combat thickening of the blood caused by liver deficiency and overeating. In the United States a billion dollars a year is spent on prescriptions for anticoagulant drugs.

---

## Hemorrhoids

Hemorrhoids are distensions of the blood veins in the anal region and therefore a form of varicose veins. These veins connect with the portal vein, which is a large vessel that goes into the liver. When the liver is congested, the movement of the blood that reaches it by way of the portal vein is obstructed. It does not manage to travel through the liver as quickly as it optimally should, and it travels in insufficient quantity, so blood begins to accumulate in the portal vein. Among other consequences, this congested state exerts pressure on the anal veins, which forces them to expand and distend.

Added to this can be the pressure that the anal veins suffer when someone pushes to evacuate hard stools. This is common during constipation, a health problem that often accompanies liver deficiency.

It stands to reason, then, that one of the basic treatments for hemorrhoids is the decongestion of the liver.

### Headaches, Migraines

Some headaches and migraines are caused by the distension of the blood vessels in the brain, which creates painful compression of the surrounding tissues.

This distension of the blood vessels is a defensive reaction to irritating and aggressive substances being transported by the bloodstream. These substances would not normally make their way into the brain at all if the liver were functioning well. A great many headaches are due to a deficiency in liver function.

This is particularly likely for migraines, which are often accompanied by nausea and vomiting.

---

### ⚠ Caution!

While taking pain relievers does offer momentary relief for headaches, their effect over the long term is counterproductive and self-defeating; by overloading the liver, they reduce its ability to neutralize irritating substances.

---

### *Other Organs*

Even organs that are farther away from the liver can suffer the consequences of hepatic deficiency.

Among its other roles, the liver has the task of filtering colloidal wastes that come from foods that are rich in starch and fat. These foods include grains and their by-products (such as bread, pasta, and cake), meat, cheese, butter, cream, and so forth.

Normally the liver removes these wastes from the bloodstream and expels them into the bile so they can be eliminated from the body with the stools. When a shortfall in liver function prevents this filtration, the wastes remain in the bloodstream and emerge from the liver by means of the hepatic vein. This allows them to move into general circulation and accumulate in the body's cellular terrain.

However, the body can intelligently defend itself against the accumulation of these toxins. If one excretory organ (in this case, the liver) is incapable of funneling the entire toxin load, the body will direct it toward other organs of elimination. Now the lungs and sebaceous glands take up the task of eliminating whatever toxins the liver was unable to filter. When toxins are too abundant, these organs will, in turn, also become exhausted and congested. Two common health problems that often result from this situation are an elimination of phlegm by the respiratory tract and acne.

## Respiratory Diseases (Catarrhal Inflammations)

Wastes that have not been filtered out of the bloodstream by the liver find their way to the lungs, bronchial tubes, or sinuses. Their presence in these organs is not normal. It leads to an inflammation of their mucous membranes, sometimes accompanied by a fever. To defend themselves, the membranes secrete a protective mucus that combines with the colloidal wastes that need to be eliminated. The result is a heavy elimination of phlegm (catarrh), as is the case in colds, sinusitis, bronchitis, and certain kinds of asthma.

While different forms of treatment for the respiratory tract can offer relief, it is primarily the restoration of normal liver function that will have a lasting healing effect. Once proper liver function has been restored, the wastes it will now be able to process will no longer make their way into the respiratory tract.

### Acne

The sebaceous glands in the skin are continuously releasing sebum, an oily matter that lubricates the skin. Sebum contains toxins of the same kind as those filtered by the liver, and as noted above, the sebaceous glands pick up some of the slack when the liver is overwhelmed by a surplus of wastes. These surplus toxins are added to the normal elimination of colloidal wastes by the sebaceous glands, and if they become overwhelmed they get congested and inflamed, at which point acne develops.

Hormonal changes in adolescence are often cited as the cause of acne, but liver deficiency also plays a role. A good cleansing of the liver is therefore strongly indicated in the treatment of acne.

---

### Colloidal Wastes

These wastes are soft and viscous, like phlegm that is expectorated or coughed out and pus that oozes out of pimples.

They are the exact opposite of the hard and insoluble crystalline waste that also is manufactured by the body. Examples of crystalline waste include grit-like crystals of uric acid that accumulate in the joints or crystals that form kidney stones.

## *Metabolic Disorders*

The accumulation of toxins in the body that follows any shortfall in normal liver function can also lead to metabolic disorders, such as those related to sugar or fat.

### Hypoglycemia Attacks

Some people are subject to recurring attacks of hypoglycemia (low blood sugar levels). They suddenly feel as if they are lacking all strength and vitality, and an overwhelming feeling of fatigue steals over them, often accompanied by dizzy spells and lightheadedness. Sometimes they feel worried and anxious. This lack of energy is due to a lack of sugar in the blood. This triggers compelling and repeated desires for sweet foods, such as chocolate, pastries, and so on.

---

### ? Did You Know?

Drinking alcohol, especially on an empty stomach, can block your liver from releasing stored glucose into your bloodstream, causing hypoglycemia and triggering a repeated desire for more alcohol or sweet foods.

---

The principal cause of hypoglycemia is the excessive consumption of bad sugars, but the liver may also be responsible. The act of going about our daily tasks "burns" blood glucose. Its content in the blood will shrink but normally we don't notice it. The liver, in its great wisdom, immediately corrects the blood sugar rate that has fallen too low and restores it to normal. It does this by releasing glucose, which it has stored for this purpose in the form of glycogen, into the bloodstream.

However, when the liver is depleted, the reconversion of

glycogen into glucose does not occur properly. The blood sugar level therefore falls below normal without the liver able to do anything to correct it, and hence the lack of energy people feel in this situation.

The solution is, consequently, detoxification of the liver. Once it has been decongested and strengthened, it will again be able to control blood sugar levels efficiently.

### Overweight

An overworked and weakened liver is one of the primary causes of obesity. Indeed, fats coming from the digestive tract pass through the liver before they even reach the tissues.

Normally the liver allows only fats that are useful to the body to pass into the bloodstream. It transforms the rest into cholesterol so it can be expelled into the bile and eliminated with the stool. Under these circumstances there is no weight gain, because no excess fats are being sent into the tissues.

Conversely, when the liver is weakened, it cannot transform those excess fats that are of no use to the body into cholesterol, or can do so only in very small quantities. The excess fats remain in the bloodstream and then enter the tissues. Their accumulation in this area will be proportionate to how much fat the liver cannot deal with and how high the fat content of the individual's diet is.

The liver is therefore the great regulator of fats. This explains why diets are not always as effective as they could be. When dietary restrictions reduce the intake of fat that the liver will need to treat, they increase the quantity of fats freed from the tissues to be burned off and used, among other things, to provide energy. However, dieting does not automatically improve the ability of a weakened and overworked liver to handle these released excess fats.

For this reason it often happens that the person following the diet makes great efforts to stick to it but has little success because the liver is not complying. It is not able to eliminate the surplus fats.

All diets intended for weight loss should therefore be accompanied by a good detoxification of the liver to support it in its job of managing fats.

### The Immune System

The deficiencies of the liver can be so pronounced that the quantity of unfiltered toxins it allows to pass through will eventually disrupt proper functioning of the entire immune system. This can be the source of a variety of problems and illnesses.

### Cancer

The majority of cancers are due to toxic substances that alter the genetic code of the cells in a harmful way. Cells then begin to multiply in a disorganized fashion and form tumors. The role of toxic substances in the proliferation of cancers has resulted in their being labeled as carcinogenic or mutagenic substances.

The most common are:

* Alcohol in excess
* Arsenic and cyanide (from cigarettes)
* Methylxanthine from coffee, tea, cola drinks, and cocoa
* Tars in grilled foods (and also in roasted coffee)
* Benzo[a]pyrene in smoked foods (meat, fish)
* Certain chemical food additives
* Mycotoxins of the molds that develop on beans and grains that have been stored improperly
* Nitrosamines (nitrates) contained in excessive amounts in

the drinking water of certain regions, as well as in some foods (particularly processed meat) and cosmetics

• Heavy metals from pollution
• Certain medications

This list is surprisingly similar to the list of harmful substances in the liver's job description. A liver that functions well is one of the fundamental elements of the battle against cancer, because it is capable of neutralizing the mutagenic substances that trigger the formation of cancerous tumors.

Its action is not only preventive, by the way, but also healing. In fact, its powerful detoxifying abilities free the cellular terrain of overloads of toxins that support the development of tumors.

The fact that the liver can be a key organ in the fight against cancer has been recognized by some researchers, but still not enough, given the great potential benefits of a regenerative treatment of the liver.

*Cancer results from a growing, chronic deficiency of the liver.*

Renowned cancer surgeon
Kasper Blond, M.D., Austria

## Autoimmune Diseases

In these increasingly common diseases (polyarthritis, lupus erythematosus, and so on), the immune system destroys the cells of the body it is designed to protect. What causes this?

When a person ingests large quantities of foods containing chemical additives, pollutants, and a variety of other toxic substances, these substances collect in the tissues, which is to say in the cells of the skin, the muscles, the skeleton, and so forth. Because they are now full of destructive substances, the immune system no longer perceives these cells as normal cells forming part of the body but as invasive and dangerous cells. It then turns against them and tries to destroy them.

The best treatment for these diseases involves the restoration of normal liver function that prevents cells from collecting so many toxic substances.

The immune system protects the body by destroying whatever attacks it. The liver stops aggressive substances from entering farther into the body. *In this way a healthy liver protects the immune system.* So it seems obvious that, as the "Liver Doctor" Sandra Cabot explains, "Diseases of the immune system are always aggravated by everything that fatigues or damages the liver." That's where it starts in the body.

## Allergies

An allergic reaction is the immune system unleashing an exaggerated histamine response to a substance not actually posing any danger to the body. This substance is not a germ or something toxic but an otherwise inoffensive substance such as an airborne irritant (pollen, dust), a kind of food (fermented foods, alcohol, cheese, and so on), or insect venom. People who are prone to allergic reactions generally metabolize histamine poorly and have trouble using and eliminating it.

The way the process works is that an allergen enters the body, either by mouth, skin, or lungs. The immune system identifies it as potentially dangerous and mobilizes antibodies to attack it. The antibodies cause the release of histamine (inflammatory chemicals) to trigger the body's defense system. However, the histamine also increases inflammation, so once it has been used for defense purposes, it should be neutralized and eliminated. This process can take place directly in the tissues or in the gut but is also a function performed by the liver.

If the histamine is not neutralized and eliminated, it lies stagnant in the tissues, which keeps the body in a pre-inflammatory and hyperreactive state. Symptoms of this can include congestion, rash, shortness of breath, coughing, and so on.

The hyperreactivity of the immune system can also be caused by the attack and irritation of the body by toxins in general, which the liver should neutralize and eliminate.

This is why a good detoxification of the liver is the exact right treatment to pursue when dealing with any form of allergy, whether it is hay fever, bronchial asthma, hives, rash, angioedema (Quincke's edema), or an allergy affecting the digestive tract.

---

### Summary

- The diseases of the liver are liver deficiency, bile stones (or gallstones), hepatitis (A, B, or C), and cirrhosis.
- The diseases resulting from poor liver function are many: indigestion, constipation, high cholesterol, cardiovascular diseases (thick blood, high blood pressure, heart attacks, strokes), hemorrhoids, headaches, migraines, catarrhs of the respiratory tract, low blood sugar, obesity, cancer, auto-immune diseases, allergies, and so on.

---

# PART 2

• • • • • •

# *How to*
# *Detoxify Your Liver*

---

## ⚠ Caution!

Various liver detoxification procedures can be used for prevention or for healing. Each is effective on its own, but it is a good idea to combine several. The one essential part of every treatment plan is reforming your diet. Unless you change your diet, it's like trying to empty a bathtub without turning off the faucet. It's a losing battle.

---

# 5

## DIETARY REFORM

Since the liver is the first organ to receive all substances that have been processed by digestion, its strength and resistance are closely dependent on what we eat.

There are three aspects to take into consideration with regard to diet in connection with the liver:

- *Foods to remove from our diet.* Some foods only exhaust the liver, attack it, or force it to overwork. It is essential to identify these foods so we can exclude them from our daily diet.
- *The dietary regime that is helpful to the liver.* We can feed ourselves in a way that is adapted to the liver's capacities. This is the diet we need to follow to support and strengthen this organ.
- *The detoxifying diet.* A restrictive diet, limited to a set period of time, will provide relief to the liver and allow it to cleanse itself of all the toxins that have been congesting it.

### FOODS TO ELIMINATE

Some foods place a heavy demand on the liver without offering much benefit to the body, and may even be harmful. The liver exhausts itself transforming and neutralizing the toxins these foods bring into the body. Eventually its capabilities become reduced and weakened, until it is no longer able to perform its work effectively.

Foods to remove from your diet include:

- Hydrogenated margarine (rich in the saturated fatty acids that are now commonly known as trans fats)
- Heat-pressed oils
- Cold cuts and sausages
- Smoked foods (fish and meat)
- Foods with high sugar content
- Food cooked in butter
- Fried foods
- Chips
- Alcohol
- Coffee and black tea
- Foods containing additives

### Bad Fats

Bad fats require the mobilization of much of the liver's strength during the digestive process, which reduces the energy it has available for detoxification. Furthermore, excess fatty acids collect in the liver and disrupt its functioning (the syndrome of congested, fatty liver).

Some people believe they are doing their livers a big favor by eliminating any consumption of fat, be it of animal or vegetable origin. However, this is not the case. If you don't include fat in your diet, your gallbladder will no longer be obliged to pour the bile it holds into the digestive tract. The bile will then lie stagnant in your gallbladder, where it will thicken and pose a greater risk of forming gallstones. In addition, because the muscles of the gallbladder are no longer working as much, they will lose their tone, which will weaken the organ.

The assimilation of liposoluble (soluble in fatty substances) vitamins such as vitamins A, D, E, and F (omega-3 and omega-6) will also be compromised. On the one hand, because these vitamins are found in fatty foods that the individual is no longer eating, they will be missing from the diet and whatever needs they fulfill in the body will go unmet. By the same token, these vitamins require bile in order to be assimilated, the bile that is precisely missing because no demand is being placed on the gallbladder, so they will still not meet the body's requirements.

In other words, while it is important to eliminate bad fats, your body needs healthy fats in order to function properly.

### An Ailing Liver and Fats

The more sick or weak the liver is, the less the individual's diet should contain animal fats, because they are high in saturated fatty acids. Fats of plant origin (virgin cold-pressed oils) and oleaginous nuts and seeds are rich in unsaturated fatty acids. The liver can tolerate fats of this origin much more easily, but quantities should be adapted to the individual's capacity.

### Excess of White Sugar and Sweets

Eating excessive amounts of sweets, especially those made with white sugar, is harmful to the liver, as all unnecessary sugar is transformed into fat and cholesterol that stagnates in the liver and bloodstream.

## *Alcohol, Food Additives, and Smoked Foods*

These foods exhaust the liver, as it is this organ's responsibility to neutralize the toxins they contain.

## *Tobacco, Drugs, and Medications*

These substances are not food per se, but they are substances that we ingest and are harmful to the liver.

### Enemies of the Liver

- Alcohol in excess: 95 percent of the alcohol ingested by the body is neutralized by the liver.
- Cigarettes: they contain many toxic substances (nicotine, arsenic, formaldehyde, and so on).
- Medications: many medicines are damaging to liver cells, particularly analgesics, hormones, antibiotics, and anti-inflammatories; these medications should only be taken when their use is absolutely essential.
- Drugs: heroin, cocaine, and so on.
- Chemical pollutants: food additives, agricultural chemicals, heavy metals from pollution, solvents, paints, and so forth.
- Overeating in general: it overworks the liver.
- Excessive fat in the diet: fatty meats, cold cuts, pâtés, sausages, fried foods, foods sautéed in butter, hydrogenated margarine.
- White sugar and sweet foods: all excess sugar ingested by the body will be converted into fat.
- Smoked foods: fish, meats.

## THE LIVER-FRIENDLY DIET

The diet that is beneficial for the liver is one that not only does not overwork it at the digestive level but also does not produce toxins that this organ cannot easily neutralize and eliminate. Another characteristic of this diet is that it supplies the liver with many nutrients that help optimize its function.

Foods that form part of this liver-friendly diet are divided into three groups. All are intrinsically beneficial, but not in just any quantity. Some can be consumed as desired, whereas others should be eaten in more modest amounts because they demand more of the liver. Then there are some that should be eaten in quite restricted quantities because of the much heavier demand they place on the liver. They nevertheless are included in this diet plan because they supply essential nutrients, such as proteins, to the body and to the liver.

### EAT AS MUCH AS YOU DESIRE

- Raw and cooked vegetables
- Raw fruits
- Germinated grains
- Water and herb tea
- Unsweetened fruit and vegetable juices
- Herbs and spices (excluding chili pepper flakes)

### EAT IN MODERATION

- Nuts
- Small seeds: sunflower, flax, pumpkin and other squash
- Starches: potatoes, rice, chestnuts
- Whole grains
- Bread, crackers, and pasta made from whole-grain flour

### EAT IN SMALL QUANTITIES

- Meat
- Fish
- Dairy products
- Eggs
- Cold-pressed plant oils
- Sweeteners: honey, maple syrup, pear and other fruit syrups without added sugar or fructose

It is preferable to prioritize fruits and vegetables that have been grown organically, as well as dairy products, eggs, and meat of free-range animals that have been fed an organic diet, as these foods will be free of toxic chemicals (herbicides, pesticides, growth hormone, antibiotics) and their ingestion will be gentler on the liver, as well as on the environment. Choose whole foods as much as possible, rather than refined foods, because they supply more of the nutrients the liver requires.

It is also extremely important to cook "light," which is to say with a minimum of fat (boiled, steamed, baked).

## THE DETOXIFYING DIET

The removal of foods that are contraindicated and the adoption of a diet that is favorable to the organ's requirements will permit the liver to gradually recover its strength and restore its health. This restoration will take a certain amount of time, however. To accelerate the detoxification of the liver, you can follow a more restrictive diet.*

---

*For a more in-depth approach, please see my books *The Detox Mono Diet: The Miracle Grape Cure and Other Cleansing Diets* (Healing Arts Press, 2006) and *Optimal Detox: How to Cleanse Your Body of Colloidal and Crystalline Toxins* (Healing Arts Press, 2013).

Indeed, when we make fewer demands on the liver in the digestive process, it can use its strength to get rid of toxins that have accumulated in it. Instead of dealing with incoming toxins, it only has to deal with congested residue. This greatly accelerates the detoxification process.

There are countless possibilities for a restrictive diet of this nature, as a diet is restrictive as soon as someone eats less than he or she usually does. More restrictive means quicker results, but it is also harder to stick with it, both physically and psychologically, as it involves more deprivation.

---

### ✛ Tips and Tricks

A balanced diet consists of:

⅔ salads and vegetables

⅓ starches and proteins

---

### *How It Works*

The diet I am suggesting here is moderately restrictive and should be able to fit anyone's needs. It is simply eating nothing but vegetables and fruits over a period from one to three days. The vegetables can be eaten raw, cooked, or juiced. Homemade vegetable soups offer another possibility. Cooked vegetables should be steamed, boiled, or baked (without oil). Fruits are also to be consumed raw, cooked, or in the form of juice. No sugar should be added to any of these, but juices can be diluted with water if you prefer.

The digestion vacation will allow the liver to cleanse itself of toxins. If, at the end of the first day of this diet, you feel great, full of pep and joy for life with no signs of exhaustion, you should continue for a second and even a third day. This diet will be even more effective if it is used in tandem with medicinal

# JOURNAL OF YOUR HABITS

To track your daily progress, note the composition of your meals in the chart below.

| | Day 1 (diet) | Day 2 (diet) | Day 3 (diet) | Day 4 | Day 5 | Day 6 | Day 7 |
|---|---|---|---|---|---|---|---|
| **Breakfast** | | | | | | | |
| **Morning snack** | | | | | | | |
| **Lunch** | | | | | | | |
| **Afternoon snack** | | | | | | | |
| **Dinner** | | | | | | | |
| **Evening snack** | | | | | | | |

plants, application of a hot-water bottle, or various other liver-stimulating methods that will be described in chapter 7.

This treatment can be repeated one or two times a month.

## HOW VITAMINS CAN HELP

The liver needs an optimum level of nutrition to support all its activities. It particularly needs vitamins and trace elements to activate the many enzymes responsible for biochemical transformations. This need intensifies when the amount of toxins is high and toxic substances are extremely aggressive (for more details, refer back to chapter 3). A generous supply of vitamins and amino acids is essential to regenerate the hepatocytes and Kupffer cells and strengthen their ability to resist the attacks of foreign substances.

Our daily diet supplies the liver with a portion of the nutrients it requires, but if the liver is sluggish or diseased, these supplies will be insufficient. Moreover, the nutritional needs of a congested liver or one with compromised ability to function are much higher. Natural food supplements, which are concentrates of vitamins, trace elements, minerals, and amino acids, are an easily absorbable way to supply the additional nutrients the liver needs at this time.

Studies have shown that the nutrients the liver needs most are vitamins from the B family and sulfur-containing amino acids such as methionine.

Natural food supplements that are rich in these substances include:

- ◆ Brewer's yeast
- ◆ Wheat germ
- ◆ Bee pollen

---

## ⚠ Caution!

Brewer's yeast is contraindicated for those susceptible to or suffering from candida or yeast infection, as it is likely to aggravate symptoms.

---

### Brewer's Yeast

Yeast molds are microscopic, single-celled fungi, so microscopic that it takes seven billion to obtain 1 gram of yeast. They are cultivated on a nutritive support substance. Brewer's yeast cultivation generally uses sprouted barley and hops.

Brewer's yeast is comprised of 50 percent amino acids, one of which is methionine. It also has a high content of B vitamins.

Brewer's yeast and wheat germ are the richest sources of B vitamins offered by nature. Generally speaking, not too many foods contain more than a few of the twelve vitamins in the B family. Brewer's yeast, however, possesses all of them, which is particularly advantageous as these vitamins work in synergy with each other, mutually supporting their individual benefits.

Brewer's yeast can be taken as powder (flakes), tablets, or liquid. The liquid form is living yeast and is thus more effective than dried yeast.

#### Dosage

*Powder:* 1 to 2 tablespoons a day, sprinkled over foods after cooking or mixed into salad dressing or yogurt. You can also drink it blended with water, with fruit or vegetable juice, or in a smoothie.

*Tablets:* Tablet size and strength varies from one manufacturer to the next, so follow the dosage directions on the package.

*Liquid:* Follow the manufacturer's instructions.

The length of time for treatment depends on the level of deficiency but should be at least two months. It is a good idea to repeat the protocol once or twice a year.

## *Wheat Germ*

Wheat germ is very high in healthy fats and other nutrients because it is the embryo of the future wheat plant and contains all the materials necessary for the first stages of the growth of the plant. It is particularly rich in all twelve of the B vitamins. Its B content is slightly lower than that of brewer's yeast, but its pleasant flavor makes it a palatable dietary staple. Wheat germ is also quite rich in vitamin E, which protects the liver and helps it regenerate. Wheat germ comes in small, gold-tinged flakes that are slightly crunchy.

### Dosage

The flakes can be blended with water, vegetable juice, cereal, yogurt, salad dressing, vegetables, or whatever else you find appealing.

The recommended dosage is 50 grams a day, which amounts to 3 to 4 tablespoons of flakes. Wheat germ can be highly stimulating, so sensitive people are advised to limit themselves to 1 to 2 tablespoons of the flakes or opt for a cycle of brewer's yeast. The remedy generally lasts for two to three months and should be repeated as needed.

---

### ✛ Tips and Tricks

Instead of buying wheat germ, you can sprout wheat seeds (1 tablespoon a day) on a plate or in a seed sprouter. When the seed sprouts in three to five days, you can eat both the sprout and the seed from which it sprouted.

---

## *Bee Pollen*

Bee pollen is the male seed of flowering plants. It is visible in the calyx of the flower as a golden powder. Bees are primarily known for harvesting the nectar they use to make honey. However, an average colony may bring in more than a hundred pounds of pollen in a season but only half that much nectar. Pollen is essential nutrition for bees as it is 40 percent protein and packed with amino acids.

Pollen contains all eight essential amino acids, but one in particular is present in noticeably high quantity: methionine. Pollen contains 3.5 grams of methionine for every 100 grams. It is the high quantity of methionine that makes bee pollen such a powerful liver cleanser.

### ? **Did You Know?**

Pure methionine is available commercially as a food supplement. Once it has been ingested and assimilated by the body, it is converted into the amino acid cysteine, a precursor of glutathione, which is a very effective detoxifier of the liver.

There are many brands of methionine available as a food supplement. The content of the gel caps varies, so follow instructions on the package to ensure you are taking the proper dose.

### Dosage

Pollen comes in the form of tiny balls (visible on the feet of bees) or tablets.

The dosage is 2 to 3 tablespoons a day. However, pollen can be highly stimulating, so you may want to start with, and possibly maintain, a smaller dose.

For those who can tolerate its very distinctive flavor, pollen balls should be well chewed and mixed with a generous amount of saliva. For others (the majority of us), it can be mixed with fruit juice or incorporated into foods. The treatment should last from one to three months.

### Sulfur

Since long ago, sulfur has been used to treat liver disorders. Modern studies have revealed the nature of sulfur's action on the liver.

Sulfur is beneficial for the liver because it:

*Stimulates the production of bile by the hepatocytes.* If hepatocytes do not receive a sufficient quantity of sulfur, their functioning slows and the liver's ability to filter and eliminate toxins and toxic substances is reduced. Conversely, their functioning is normal provided they are supplied with sufficient sulfur, and increasing sulfur can intensify their effectiveness.

*Activates numerous enzymes that play a role in detoxification.* Enzymes are responsible for all the biochemical transformations the body needs to function and to cleanse itself. They have the capacity to achieve an enormous amount of work, but in order to perform their tasks, they must be activated, or in other words, stimulated. Sulfur is the primary catalyst for this starting impulse for liver enzymes. Without sulfur, the biochemical transformations necessary for the neutralization and elimination of toxins will not be made or will be inadequate.

*Neutralizes heavy metals.* Heavy metals such as lead, mercury, cadmium, and so forth are poison for the body. Thanks to sulfur, the liver deactivates their toxic properties. This neutralization is beneficial not only because it prevents the body from having to suffer the attacks of these toxic substances, but also because it facilitates their evacuation from the tissues, and ultimately from the body.

*Forms part of the composition of four amino acids (methionine, cysteine, taurine, and homocysteine) that are necessary for the liver to detoxify and regenerate.* These sulfur-containing amino acids combine with and neutralize toxic substances so they can be eliminated.

*Encourages oxygenation of the liver.* Like all the other cells of the body, the cells of the liver can only work if they are well oxygenated. Sulfur is an important nutrient in this oxygenation.

## Foods Rich in Sulfur

Numerous foods contain sulfur. Stark deficiencies in this mineral are, therefore, rare. However, increasing the amount of sulfur available to the liver intensifies its functionality and encourages detoxification.

The following table presents foods with particularly high sulfur content.

## FOODS WITH HIGH SULFUR CONTENT

| Foods | Sulfur Content (in milligrams per 100 grams) |
|---|---|
| **Animal Products** | |
| Fowl | 230–280 |
| Eggs | 188 |
| Seafood | 180–370 |
| Red meat | 140–250 |
| Fish | 130–290 |
| **Cruciferous Vegetables (cabbage family)** | |
| Broccoli | 137 |
| Brussels sprouts | 80 |
| White and green cabbage | 70 |
| Red cabbage | 68 |

| Foods | Sulfur Content (in milligrams per 100 grams) |
|---|---|
| **Alliaceous Vegetables (garlic family)** | |
| Leeks | 72 |
| Chives | 49 |
| Garlic, shallots, onions | 34 |
| **Vegetables** | |
| Green beans | 220 |
| Horseradish | 212 |
| Lamb's lettuce (*Valerianella locusta*) | 200 |
| Parsley | 190 |
| Dried peas | 174 |
| Watercress | 147 |
| Lettuce | 60 |
| Corn | 57 |
| Green peas | 55 |
| Radishes | 39 |
| Turnips | 34 |
| Potatoes | 30 |
| Spinach | 29 |
| **Fruits and Nuts** | |
| Avocados | 225 |
| Brazil nuts, hazelnuts | 198 |
| Walnuts | 180 |
| Almonds | 155 |
| Peaches | 140 |
| Apricots | 100 |

## Sulfuric Mineral Water

Certain mineral waters are high in sulfur and for this reason are recommended for invigorating the liver. Regular intake of these waters as a table beverage and between meals, from 1 to 1.5 liters a day, will help the liver detoxify. Treatment lasts a minimum of one to two months.

### MINERAL WATERS CONTAINING SULFUR

| | |
|---|---|
| San Pellegrino | 445 mg/l |
| Vittel | 337 mg/l |
| Vichy-Célestin | 138 mg/l |
| Calistoga Sparkling | 110 mg/l |
| Perrier | 46 mg/l |
| Gerolsteiner | 38 mg/l |
| Crystal Geyser | 36 mg/l |

## Trace Element: Sulfur

Sulfur can also be taken as a trace element. In this form, the quantity of sulfur is extremely reduced. So what we are dealing with here is a supply based not on quantity but on quality. Sulfur taken as a trace element doesn't just serve as a catalyst for the enzymes that detoxify the liver, it also encourages the incorporation of the sulfur ingested by the body in food and mineral water.

The trace element remedy comes in the form of a liquid that contains sulfur. The small bottle that contains the liquid is generally accompanied by a measuring spoon, or has a device to give a dose. The customary dosage is 1 measuring spoon a day. In order to support its assimilation, the liquid should be ingested on an empty stomach before eating breakfast in the morning. Hold it under your tongue for one minute to facilitate absorption into the mouth's blood vessels. In this way it will be made available to the entire body right away.

---

### ✛ Tips and Tricks

Take 1 measuring spoon of sulfur trace element liquid in the morning on an empty stomach. Hold beneath the tongue for one minute before swallowing.

---

Taking the trace element form of sulfur can trigger reactions such as nausea and diarrhea, so it's a good idea to start treatment by taking one dose every three days, in order to observe how your liver reacts. In the absence of any problems, gradually increase the frequency to once every two days, then up to once a day.

If your reactions are strong, it's better to stop taking the trace element and consume sulfur in food or beverages.

A full treatment lasts from two to four months.

---

### In Practice

- Be wary of fats, sugar, and alcohol, all of which exhaust the liver.
- Count on fruits and vegetables, which stimulate the work of the liver.
- The liver's requirements for nutrients are quite high. Three food supplements are especially recommended: brewer's yeast, wheat germ, and bee pollen.
- Sulfur promotes detoxification by the liver. There are three ways in which you can take sulfur: certain foods, mineral waters, or trace elements.

---

# 6

# Medicinal Plants for Liver Health

Phytotherapy is one of the most effective means of stimulating liver function. Medicinal plants used for a liver purge are called "hepatic plants" or "liver drainers."

## THE ACTION OF HEPATIC PLANTS

Hepatic plants work in three different ways:

### Choleretic Action

These plants stimulate the hepatocytes to produce more bile. In a best-case scenario, the output can double, which is advantageous not only for better digestion but also because a greater quantity of bile means a greater quantity of toxins and toxic substances being eliminated from the body. The principal choleretic plants are artichoke, alder buckthorn, milk thistle, celandine, chicory, turmeric, dandelion, yellow gentian, rosemary, and goldenrod.

### Cholagogue Action

These plants act first and foremost to tone and stimulate the muscles of the walls of the gallbladder, increasing the organ's ability to contract and eject bile. This results in an increase in the quantity of bile available for digestion and of toxins being eliminated. It also greatly reduces the risks of gallstones forming. The main cholagogue plants are artichoke, boldo (leaves from a tree that grows in Chile), common barberry, common polypody (a type of fern), and black radish.

### Protective Action

These plants protect hepatocytes from attack. The mission of the cells of the liver is to neutralize toxic substances that are dangerous to the body, but they are also vulnerable to attack by these toxic substances. Fortunately, nature provides plants that offer protection against such assaults, known as hepatoprotective plants.

They act in the following way:

- They halt the penetration of toxic substances into the hepatocytes by increasing the resistant quality of their membranes. Normally toxic substances, the hepatitis virus, alcohol, and so on do not enter the hepatocytes but remain outside (in the perisinusoidal space, or space of Disse) to be neutralized. However, because of their aggressive nature, some toxic substances can injure the cellular membrane and invade the cell. The damage caused by these intruders then prevents the hepatocytes from performing their work, or damages and kills a quantity of liver cells. Hepatoprotective plants work to avoid or minimize this aggression.
- They increase the production of molecules and enzymes that the liver uses to destroy toxic substances. These latter are thereby more quickly and efficiently neutralized, which also helps spare the liver from their harmful effects.

- They stimulate the regeneration of injured cells by promoting the synthesis of proteins needed to heal and reactivate them, hastening the process.
- They stimulate the replacement of cells, thus maintaining the liver in an optimum state of functioning.

The principal hepatoprotective plants known today include milk thistle, chrysanthellum, and desmodium (or tick clover).

The hepatoprotective plants are especially recommended for anyone whose liver has suffered from ingestion of medications, drugs, or excessive alcohol or who has endured hepatitis, chemical poisoning, or other forms of poisoning.

The choleretic, cholagogue, and hepatoprotective properties are present in different proportions in the different plants. No plant is exclusively choleretic or cholagogue; both properties are always present, but one takes precedence over the other. Hepatoprotective properties, on the other hand, are much more rare; we know of only a small number of hepatic plants endowed with these properties.

### How to Dose with Hepatic Plants

To obtain a broad and permeating effect on the liver, it is a good idea to take hepatic plants three times a day, before meals. In this way its work will be stimulated and supported three times every day. Over time these regular, repeated ingestions will help the liver gradually decongest itself of encumbering wastes. It will strengthen itself, recover normal functioning, and start working more intensively.

### Length of Treatment

The congestion of the liver by wastes and its resulting weakening is a process that takes place over a prolonged period of time. Years of gradual poisoning obviously cannot be undone with a few days of treatment. Practice has shown that while beneficial effects will begin to appear in several days of a remedy, the treatment must extend over a period of two to three months if you want profound effects. At that time you can take a break of one to two months and then start the treatment again. One to two rounds a year should maintain the liver in its proper functioning state.

---

### ✪ Tips and Tricks

Start with a treatment cycle of six weeks. Every two weeks change the plant you are using in order to gain more experience in the use of hepatic plants. Over time you will discover which plants are best suited for you.

---

### *Dosage*

The dosages suggested for hepatic plants are average doses that should be adapted to each individual, as reactions will vary from one individual to the next. For some people the average dose is too low; for others it's too high.

The goal is to take as much as needed to obtain good results, but without this effect being too pronounced and inconveniencing you. The effect of taking hepatic plants is observed not directly on the liver, but indirectly on the intestines, where the increased volume of bile secretion triggered by the plant has laxative effects. The stools become more watery, and instead of taking place once a day, elimination occurs two or three times daily. The correct dosage is therefore the one that is the highest possible without causing too strong a laxative effect.

It is recommended that you begin by taking less than the average dose, then increasing it every day until you experience a slight laxative effect, which indicates the appropriate dosage for you.

## NINE HIGHLY
## EFFECTIVE PLANTS
## FOR DETOXIFYING THE LIVER

Each of these plants is beneficial, but each has slightly different action, so it is preferable to change plants over the course of a long treatment. This also ensures that the body does not become accustomed to one particular plant and have a diminished reaction to it.

---

### ✪ Tips and Tricks

*Mother tinctures:* This remedy is obtained by macerating the plant matter in alcohol in a precise ratio of 10 percent plant matter to 90 percent alcohol.

*Herbal teas:* A large number of "liver-gallbladder" or "hepatic" teas, made from a blend of plants with complementary hepatic properties, are available for general purchase. Consult your local herbalist or health food store specialist for specific recommendations.

---

The following nine plants are highly effective at cleansing the liver.

### Artichoke *(Cynara scolymus)*
The part used in therapy is not the bud of the flower but the leaves. They stimulate the production of bile effectively but

gently, hence their popularity as a liver cleanser. Artichoke leaves are especially recommended for children and the elderly. They also have slightly diuretic properties.

*Infusion:* 5 tablespoons of leaves per liter of water, let steep for ten minutes, drink three cups a day. This is a very bitter drink.

*Gel caps:* 1 or 2 capsules, three times daily.

*Mother tincture:* 20 to 30 drops, three times a day.

### Milk Thistle *(Silybum marianum)*

This plant belongs to the thistle family. Its flowers are a violet-purple and its leaves are fringed with thorns. Generally the leaves are used for their stimulating properties on the production and transit of bile, but in addition, recent studies have shown that the seeds of milk thistle contain silymarin, a hepatoprotective substance.

*Infusion:* 1 to 2 teaspoons of the plant per cup, let steep for ten minutes, drink three cups a day.

*Gel caps:* 1 or 2 capsules, three times daily.

*Mother tincture:* 20 to 30 drops, three times a day.

### Chrysanthellum *(Chrysanthellum americanum)*

This grass-like plant is traditionally used in South America to detoxify the liver, and it has recently been revealed as having hepatoprotective properties.

*Decoction:* 5 heaping tablespoons per ¾ liter of water, boil gently for ten minutes, drink three times a day.

*Gel caps:* 1 or 2 capsules, three times daily.

*Mother tincture:* 30 to 50 drops, three times a day.

## Dandelion *(Taraxacum officinale)*

This well-known plant enlivens lawns and meadows with its bright yellow flowers. It takes its name from its long, serrated leaves; in French, *dent de lion* (pronounced don-de-leeon) means lion's tooth. It stimulates all the functions of the liver, which means both the production and elimination of bile, and is considered by many herbalists to be one of the best plants with hepatic properties. The use of dandelion greens in salad is highly recommended.

*Infusion:* One large handful of dried leaves and roots per liter of water, boil for two minutes, then let steep for ten minutes. Drink three cups a day.

*Gel caps:* 1 or 2 capsules, three times daily.

*Mother tincture:* 30 to 50 drops, three times a day.

## Desmodium *(Desmodium adscendens)*

A creeping plant of the Leguminosae family that grows in the moist areas of tropical regions, desmodium has a pronounced protective and regulating effect on the liver.

*Infusion:* 1 tablespoon of the dried plant per 10 ounces of water, boil for two minutes, then let steep for ten minutes. Drink three cups a day.

*Mother tincture:* 30 to 50 drops, three times a day.

## Common Fumitory *(Fumaria officinalis)*

The flowering tops of this plant, nicknamed the "jaundice plant," are excellent regulators of all hepatic functions.

*Infusion:* One large handful of flowering tops per liter of water, let steep for ten minutes, drink three cups a day.

*Gel caps:* 1 or 2 capsules, three times daily.
*Mother tincture:* 10 to 20 drops, three times a day.

### Black Radish *(Raphanus sativus)*

This long radish has a narrow tip at one end and can grow to 8 inches in length. Its flesh is white, but contrary to other radishes, its skin is not red or pink but black. It has the spicy, sulfurous flavor typical of radishes. Black radish is an excellent liver stimulant, but its primary effect is on the gallbladder (cholagogic effect). Its use in cooking is highly recommended.

*Vial of black radish juice:* 1 to 3 vials a day according to manufacturer's instructions.
*Gel caps:* 1 or 2 capsules, three times daily.
*Mother tincture:* 30 to 40 drops, three times a day.

### Rosemary *(Rosmarinus officinalis)*

A shrub native to the regions of the Mediterranean, rosemary grows in stems of multiple small narrow leaves that have powerful choleretic (they can double bile production) and cholagogic properties. Rosemary's effects are so powerful that a treatment using this herb should be limited to one month. Rosemary also has a very stimulating and galvanizing effect, so it is not recommended for anyone with a nervous temperament. Its use in cooking is strongly recommended.

*Infusion:* 1 teaspoon of the leaves per cup, let steep for fifteen minutes, drink two to three cups a day.
*Gel caps:* 1 or 2 capsules, three times daily.
*Mother tincture:* 20 to 40 drops, three times a day.

**Goldenrod** *(Solidago virgaurea)*

The flowering tops of this plant are a very bright yellow in color; hence its popular name. This plant flowers at the end of summer. It is an excellent stimulant of hepatic functions and also has diuretic properties.

*Infusion:* One large handful of the dried plant per liter of water, boil for two minutes, then let steep for ten minutes. Drink three cups a day.

*Gel caps:* 1 or 2 capsules, three times daily.

*Mother tincture:* 30 to 40 drops, three times a day.

## TREATMENTS FOR GALLSTONES

Hepatic plants not only stimulate the liver, they also have an effect on gallstones.

The elimination of small gallstones, meaning those small enough to be able to pass through the cystic duct and the bile duct, can be managed with the use of hepatic plants with cholagogic properties.

Cholagogic plants trigger the emptying of the gallbladder. This draining action will rid the gallbladder of biliary sludge and tiny gallstones, as well as tonify the muscles of the gall-bladder's walls. When the body demands bile for digestion, the gallbladder will contract more effectively and thus empty itself more completely than before. Over time this allows it to eliminate all the sludge and tiny gallstones it has been holding.

### The Black Radish Remedy

Black radish is highly indicated for the necessary draining of the liver. The treatment consists of ingesting it every morning on an empty stomach for one to two months.

*Dosage:* 1 teaspoon (50 drops) of mother tincture of black radish blended with lemon juice. Dilute this mixture in a large
glass of water.

The lemon plays an accompanying role here. It stimulates
hepatic, gastric, and pancreatic secretions. There is no major
drawback to not taking it, and it should be avoided if you are
sensitive to fruit acids.

One alternative to black radish mother tincture would be
vials of black radish juice.

The cholagogic action of black radish is both gentle and
gradual. It will not trigger violent contractions of the gallbladder, which could cause the migration of large gallstones. To the
contrary, it very gently tones the muscles of the gallbladder. The
biliary sludge and tiny gallstones are thereby eliminated gradually and smoothly.

It should be noted that dandelion works in the same way
and is administered in the same manner.

### The Olive Oil Express

Another way to drain the gallbladder is with an olive oil
treatment.

When fats reach the duodenum as they exit the stomach, a
signal is sent to the gallbladder to contract. Normally this takes
place during a meal, but you can take advantage of this process
by intentionally ingesting a large quantity of fat between meals.
This will stimulate and empty the gallbladder, including whatever tiny gallstones and biliary sludge it may contain. Olive oil
has been the lubricant of choice for this task for a long time.
Make sure the olive oil you use is first cold pressed and virgin.

Two treatments are possible:

- For a period of ten to fifteen days, ingest 1 to 2 tablespoons of olive oil in the morning on an empty stomach. This treatment should be repeated several times a year.

♦ The night before starting the treatment, eat only vegetable soup or raw vegetables. The next morning before breakfast, ingest 6 to 7 tablespoons of olive oil. Half an hour later the oil will reach the duodenum and prompt an energetic draining of the gallbladder. Repeat the treatment three days in a row or once a month for three months. Warning: This method can be fairly violent. It places a strong demand on the digestive tract because of the amount of oil that has been ingested. To facilitate its digestion, try adding some lemon juice to the oil.

### Dissolving Large Gallstones

Some gallstones are too large to be able to pass through the cystic duct and the bile duct in order to reach the intestines. Simply speaking, they are wider than the diameter of these ducts. The ideal solution, therefore, would be to find a way to dissolve these gallstones. Once reduced to "dust" they could be easily carried away by the bile.

Over the course of time a variety of medicinal plants have been suggested for this task. Among them we find artichoke, boldo, birch, nettle, black radish, and so forth. Their description as dissolving plants, however, needs to be taken with a grain of salt. In fact, the proof that these plants possess this property has never been clearly demonstrated. The improvements that have been observed after the taking of these plants seems more likely to be due to the energetic draining of the gallbladder. Cleared of the biliary sludge and smaller gallstones, the organ is functioning more effectively despite the remaining presence of large gallstones.

## ⚠ Caution!

The effectiveness of the olive oil treatment can be a double-edged sword. The intense draining may carry along a large gallstone that can clog the cystic duct or the bile duct.

## In Practice

- Hepatic plants stimulate liver function in three different ways: they stimulate the production of bile, they stimulate draining of the gallbladder, and they protect liver cells against toxins.

- Thanks to a treatment adapted to the specific circumstances of the individual, the liver little by little decongests and eliminates burdensome wastes. It becomes stronger, recovers normal functioning, and starts working more intensively.

- Cholagogic plants provide conditions that are favorable for the evacuation of smaller gallstones. Two remedies are suggested: the black radish remedy or the olive oil express.

# 7

# STIMULATING THE LIVER WITH HEAT, EXERCISE, AND MASSAGE

In addition to diet and herbs, there are external ways to stimulate the liver and ensure its proper functioning.

## HOT-WATER BOTTLE

The hot-water bottle is an extremely effective method for stimulating liver function. The liver is the warmest organ in the body with a temperature that varies from 102° to 105.8°F (39°–41°C). The execution of its many functions produces a great deal of heat, so the liver is not only accustomed to working at this temperature, it needs it in order to function properly.

### Heat for the Liver
Heat loss in the hepatic gland will slow down the rate at which it performs its duties. This can occur when a person has been weakened by illness but also can result from overexertion, stress, substandard nutrition, or nutritional deficiencies, or quite simply if the individual is not dressed warmly enough for

the external temperature. When the liver drops in temperature there is a vasoconstrictive effect on its blood capillaries. Their diameter shrinks, which slows blood circulation and reduces the amount of blood they contain.

Normally the liver is particularly well supplied with blood. As we have seen, it weighs 3.3 pounds when dry and 5.5 pounds when engorged with blood. Blood, therefore, represents almost half its total weight. This blood circulates in the sinusoidal capillaries that snake between the hepatocytes. A lack of blood in the liver will hamper the filtration and elimination of wastes. This problem of a drop in temperature in the area of the liver can easily be remedied by a supply of heat that brings increased blood flow to the organ. A hot-water bottle is a very simple and effective way to do this.

*By bringing additional heat to the liver, a hot-water bottle accelerates the rate at which it functions.*

Placed over the region of the liver, the hot-water bottle will transmit heat to this organ, causing its temperature to rise. Its blood capillaries will dilate, which will automatically increase the quantity of blood present in the liver and bring it back to its normal level. It may even exceed this level during the time the hot-water bottle remains applied. The liver will emerge from its lethargy and resume functioning with pep and efficiency.

## Steps to Follow

+ *Place the bottle filled with hot water on the front of the body in the liver area.* Hot water from the tap is hot enough; water heated in a kettle will be too hot. The hot-water bottle can be placed over clothing or directly on the skin.

+ *Leave it in place for fifteen to thirty minutes.* Begin with short sessions (ten minutes), then gradually increase them up to thirty or forty-five minutes, during which time it's best to remain still, either sitting or lying down. You can move around a little, but not so much that the hot-water bottle might slip off its target.

• *Apply one to three times a day,* preferably after meals. Sessions can take place right after a meal, during a nap, in bed before going to sleep, sitting down while reading, and so on.

## EXERCISES FOR THE LIVER

Blood flow is steady, strong, and abundant in the liver—1 liter a minute out of a total of 5 liters in the body. The liver needs all this blood in order to perform its functions properly. Congestion of the liver is characterized by the stagnation of blood and wastes, and like a vicious cycle, the slowing of blood circulation fosters congestion, so the momentum of incoming blood is no longer strong enough to push along blood already in the organ. When the liver does not "empty" enough of its blood, its rate of flow can fall below 1 liter a minute. It is not receiving high-enough pressure for the filtering process to be carried out properly.

*Physical exercise is one way to remedy stagnation of the blood in the liver and its immediate surroundings.*

Physical exercise strongly accelerates blood circulation in general and therefore that of the liver as well.

---

### ⚠ Caution!

In order to be physiologically beneficial, these exercises should be introduced gradually and practiced within your physical capabilities and without exaggeration.

---

Two procedures are used here: self-massaging your liver with two bending exercises, and increasing blood flow by exercising until you are out of breath.

### Self-Massage of the Liver with Bending Exercises

The purpose of these bending exercises is to exert pressure on the liver and gallbladder in such a way that it causes the blood to drain. Because these exercises compress the blood vessels of these organs, the stagnant, waste-laden blood they contain is pushed farther into the circulatory system. The void thus created in the blood vessel is immediately filled by new, well-oxygenated blood. By repeating the movements several times, the liver is alternately compressed and decompressed. It functions the same way as a sponge that is squeezed and released several times in succession.

#### Lateral Bends of the Torso

- Begin in a standing position.
- Interlock your hands behind your head, elbows extending to either side.

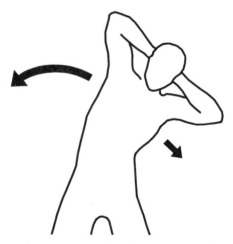

*Lateral bends of the torso*

- Remaining upright, perform lateral bends alternately to the left side, then to the right, in rhythm with your breathing.
- Breathe in when bending to the right so that your lungs full of air will squeeze the liver more effectively.
- Perform three sets of ten, twenty, or thirty bends per day, with a rest between each set.

### Forward Bends

- Begin in a seated position.
- Join your hands together at the nape of your neck, elbows extending to either side.
- Lean forward, keeping your back straight and flat as much as possible, until your torso touches your knees.
- Breathe in while bending forward; exhale as you return to the upright position.
- Perform three sets of ten, twenty, or thirty bends a day, with a rest between each set.

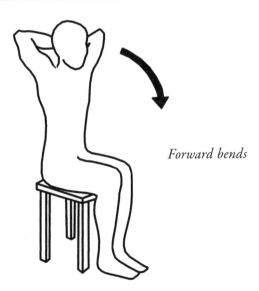

*Forward bends*

### *Increasing Blood Flow through Breathlessness*

When the liver is functioning properly, all the blood contained in the human body (5 liters) will travel through it every five minutes. However, this is not possible when the hepatic filter is congested. The restoration of normal blood flow through the liver, and even an increase in this flow, can be obtained by physical activities that cause breathlessness. Why is this necessary?

Your muscles need oxygen to work. The more intense the muscular activity, the more the body needs oxygen. To address this need, we inhale more deeply and rapidly to absorb the maximum amount of oxygen possible. This acceleration in the breath rate causes an acceleration of blood circulation, as it is the bloodstream that transports oxygen to the muscles. The muscles then receive it quickly and in large quantity. When you run out of breath and your heart pumps faster and harder, blood circulation has increased throughout the body, including, of course, to and through the liver.

The most effective way to run out of breath is to place demands on the body's largest muscle masses—the thighs. Their need for oxygen is heightened and increases quickly with exercise. The strong breathlessness that results from exercises concentrated on the thighs can double or triple the speed of the bloodstream and consequently its passage through the liver.

Different exercises might include:

#### Squats

- Stand up straight with your legs slightly apart.
- Bend your knees so as to bring your buttocks down by your heels, as if you were about to sit in a chair.
- Extend your arms forward to keep your balance.
- Once you are sitting close to your heels, start to straighten your legs and return to your original position.

- Do three sets of ten, twenty, or more bends, depending on your physical ability.
- Give yourself a chance to rest between each set.
- With practice, increase the speed with which you perform the squats—the faster you do these exercises, the more quickly you will run short of breath and the blood flow will accelerate.

## Running or Jogging

- Run at a moderate pace until you start running short of breath.
- Stop running, then walk quietly until your respiration and cardiac rhythm return to normal.
- Continue alternating walking and running several times.
- You will run out of breath more quickly on an upward trajectory than on flat terrain.

## Cycling

- Go for a bike ride (or hop on a stationary bike) and pedal at a sustained rhythm for fifteen to thirty minutes, or more, depending on your physical capability. This effort will cause a profound state of breathlessness and trigger a sharp acceleration of blood flow throughout your body, including through the liver.

The exercises presented here are not the only possible ones. In reality, any physical or athletic activity has the potential to cause you to run short of breath. If you choose one you enjoy, you are more likely to do it consistently.

## MASSAGE

### *Liver Massage*

Massage unclogs a congested liver and stimulates its functioning. However, the liver is not directly accessible to massage the way the intestines are; it lies concealed beneath the ribs, which protect it from external shocks. It can, nonetheless, be accessed in the zone located in the hollow of the stomach and above the right hip, following the edge of the ribs. By massaging the soft tissue in this area, in other words by going "in search" of the liver by slightly digging beneath the ribs with your fingers, you can have a direct effect on a small portion of this organ, with repercussions that radiate to the entire liver.

Liver massage consists of rubbing this particular zone. Lying on a firm surface will provide easier access. Using the three longest fingers on your left (or right) hand, apply circular pressure to the hepatic region. The rubbing should be gentle and superficial to start, but over time you should press deeper and more emphatically. Massage for two to three minutes on the first days, but gradually increase for up to a dozen minutes.

### Massage of the Reflex Zones on the Feet

The reflex zones on the soles of the feet are small surfaces of skin where a specific nerve emanating from one or another organ of the body terminates. Each organ of the body is connected to one of these very specific cutaneous zones on the bottom of the feet. Because of this connection, the deterioration of an organ's health will have a repercussion on its reflex zone. If the organ is ailing, this zone will become sensitive, even painful to touch. The amount of pain it engenders is proportionate to the seriousness of the disorder afflicting the organ in question.

Fortunately this connection allows the transmission of information in both directions. Massage of the reflex zone stimulates in the other direction, toward the organ to which it is connected.

This massage is done with the thumb or a knuckle. In the beginning the reflex zone should be rubbed two or three times a day for only a few minutes (two to five minutes). Later the duration of the massage can be increased up to ten or even twenty minutes. To ensure that your fingers slide easily over the surface of the reflex zone and don't irritate the skin, it is a good idea to rub oil or cream on the skin before beginning to massage it. The reflex zones for the liver and the gallbladder are located on the sole of the right foot.

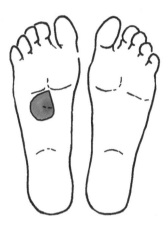

*The reflex zones of the liver*

---

### In Practice

The liver can be stimulated using several different methods:

- The liver functions at a temperature between 102° and 106°F. A hot-water bottle will raise the liver's temperature and stimulate its work.

- Exercises such as lateral and forward bends of the torso compress the liver. This increases blood circulation, which in turn activates liver function.

- Directly massaging the area of the liver or applying pressure to the liver's reflex zones on the soles of the feet stimulates liver function.

---

# 8

# TREATING THE LIVER
# VIA THE INTESTINES

You can also work indirectly on the liver by way of the intestines. In fact, when intestinal transit is normal, the time during which toxins in the stool remain in contact with intestinal mucous membranes is limited. This time of contact increases when transit slows and becomes potentially harmful, proportionate to the severity of the constipation.

Two harmful consequences of this prolonged contact are:

* A larger quantity of toxins is absorbed by the body.
* The intestinal mucous membranes are injured by the aggressive nature of the toxins, which in turn allows toxins to more easily enter the bloodstream and therefore be transported to the liver by the portal vein.

## RESTORING NORMAL INTESTINAL TRANSIT

An important step for countering these harmful effects would be to restore a normal intestinal transit and even, perhaps, one that is a little faster than normal.

A good intestinal transit reduces the quantity of toxins

that the liver must deal with because they get eliminated before they can be absorbed by the body. There are a variety of ways to achieve acceleration of the intestinal transit.

### Laxatives

A laxative is a remedy that accelerates the passage of stools through the intestine. You can achieve a good draining of the intestines by taking a medicinal plant for a week or two, such as alder buckthorn, golden shower tree (*Cassia fistula*), or mallow. Given the taste of some of these plants, it is preferable to use them in the form of mother tinctures. In this case, 15 to 50 drops three times a day should suffice. Take this with a little water before meals.

### Powdered Whey

Another way to gently stimulate the emptying of the intestines is to use whey (the liquid that escapes from coagulated milk) in the form of powder (available in most vitamin and food stores). The dosage is around 1 tablespoon of whey in ½ to 1 cup of water. Drink two to four glasses a day right before meals or between them as a snack. Increase or reduce the number of glasses of whey you drink based on how it affects you. Follow this program for one to two weeks to allow for a good emptying of the intestines.*

### High-Fiber Food Remedies

Food remedies such as flaxseed and psyllium are characterized by high fiber content in the form of mucilage. On contact with

---

*For more on the healing properties of whey, see my book *The Whey Prescription: The Healing Miracle in Milk* (Healing Arts Press, 2006).

water, these fibers expand to five and ten times their initial volume, respectively, forming a soft, voluminous, moist gel that promotes the passage of stool by stimulating peristalsis. These two food remedies do not replace a high-fiber diet (whole grains, fruits, and vegetables) so much as complement it. The choice is yours:

- *Flax seeds:* 1 to 3 tablespoons a day mixed into food or a beverage. They can also be chewed for several minutes before being swallowed. Follow with a large glass of water.
- *Psyllium:* 2 to 3 teaspoons a day of psyllium powder mixed with water. Gradually increase the dosage until you find the one that is right for you. Drink a large glass of water immediately after you have swallowed the psyllium.

### Fruits with Laxative Effects

Certain fruits vigorously stimulate the intestinal transit. A daily consumption of these kinds of fruits will thereby support the eliminatory work performed by the intestines.

- *Prunes:* Eat two or three prunes as they are or after they have been left overnight to steep in a bowl of water. Experiment with the dosage until you find the desired effect.
- *Dried figs:* Eat two or three dried figs as they are or after reconstituting them overnight in a bowl of water. Experiment with the dosage until you find the desired effect.

## In Practice

Maintaining a good intestinal transit supports the function of the liver.

To accelerate your intestinal transit and thereby offer relief to your liver, a variety of possible remedies exist:

- Laxatives
- Powdered whey
- Foods high in fiber
- Fruits with laxative properties

# 9

# TREATMENT PROTOCOLS

There are many ways to treat the liver using a variety of techniques. Through trial and error you can discover the best way for you to proceed, based on your specific needs. I am going to introduce four examples of these different treatments. Specifications will be provided in each one for the kinds of people they are targeting and what their anticipated effects will be.

---

### ⚠ Caution!

For all these treatments a change in diet is necessary. The elimination of the most harmful foods (see the discussion of foods to remove from your diet on page 66) should be sufficient for a simple remedy.

For the intensive remedies, in addition to this step you will need to follow—as much as you possibly can—a diet that is favorable for the liver (see page 70).

---

## THE SIMPLE REMEDY

### (ONE TO THREE MONTHS)

*Indications:* This treatment is indicated for those who would like to:

- Be proactive about their health
- Familiarize themselves with detoxification
- Provide relief to a liver that has been temporarily congested by dietary excess (travel or holiday indulgence, for example)

*The state of the liver:*
- Slightly congested
- In need of a modest cleansing

*Effects:* Stimulation and detoxification of the liver.

*The treatment*: Consists of two detoxification procedures. One involves taking a medicinal plant for the liver; the other is one procedure that can be selected from the options offered below.

### Medicinal Plants
- Artichoke
- Dandelion
- Black radish

Take the remedy you have selected by following the instructions provided in chapter 6.

### Supplemental Treatments
To reinforce the detoxification of the liver, top off the plant treatment above with one of the following procedures:
- Hot-water bottle, once a day in the evening (especially recommended for those who are sensitive to the cold)
- Sulfur trace element
- Reflexology massage once a day for five to ten minutes

◆ Vitamins (brewer's yeast or bee pollen), recommended for those who feel constantly fatigued and lack energy

## THE SIMPLE LONG TREATMENT
### (THREE TO SIX MONTHS)

*Indications:* This treatment is indicated for those who:
◆ Suffer regularly from digestive issues
◆ Have difficulty digesting fats and large meals

*The state of the liver:*
◆ Congested
◆ Fatigued and lazy
◆ Weak

*Effects:*
◆ Decongests the liver
◆ Activates its functioning
◆ Fortifies the liver

*The treatment:* This program consists of taking three medicinal plants in succession, combined with two other detoxification procedures.

### Medicinal Plants
Take the following herbal remedies, changing the plant every month. For example:
◆ First month: artichoke
◆ Second month: milk thistle
◆ Third month: goldenrod

Take the remedy following the instructions in chapter 6.

Take note: If your body has trouble assimilating one plant (if it causes you cramps, intestinal discomfort, and so forth), replace it with another one.

### Supplemental Treatments

As a reinforcement effort for cleansing your liver, top off the herbal treatment with the following remedies:

- Sulfurous mineral water, 1–1.5 quarts a day
- Supplements: do a cycle of brewer's yeast or bee pollen

## THE SHORT INTENSIVE TREATMENT
### (ONE TO THREE WEEKS)

Indications: This treatment is indicated for those who:

- Are overworked and stressed
- Eat too much food and too much that has poor nutritional value
- Abuse alcohol and stimulants

Condition of the liver:

- Extremely congested
- Overworked and weakened

Effects: Significant cleansing of the liver, yet it will not be fully cleansed because of the short duration of the treatment.

The treatment: This treatment consists of taking a medicinal plant combined with five detoxification procedures intended to encourage the liver to cleanse.

### *Medicinal Plants*

Choose one of the three following plants:

- Rosemary
- Dandelion
- Black radish

Take the remedy following the instructions in chapter 6.

### *Supplemental Treatments*

To reinforce the detoxifying benefits of this treatment, complete the herbal treatment with the following remedies:

- Diet: eat a generous amount of sulfurous vegetables
- Apply a hot-water bottle, three times a day
- Take a supplement of the trace element sulfur
- Reflexology massage, twice a day for five to fifteen minutes
- Supplements: brewer's yeast or bee pollen

## THE LONG INTENSIVE TREATMENT
### (ONE TO THREE MONTHS)

*Indications:* This treatment is indicated for those who:

- Suffer from chronic weakness of the liver
- Suffer from ongoing digestive problems
- Have difficulty digesting fats and large meals

*Liver condition:*

- Extremely congested
- Extremely overworked

*Effects:*
- Decongests the liver
- Fortifies the liver
- Regenerates the liver

*The treatment:* This protocol consists of taking three medicinal plants in succession, combined with five other tested detoxification techniques designed to cleanse and regenerate the liver.

### Medicinal Plants
Take the following herbal plants, changing the plant every month. For example:
- First month: dandelion
- Second month: common fumitory
- Third month: artichoke

Take the remedy following the instructions in chapter 6.

Take note: If your body has difficulty assimilating one plant (if you experience cramps, intestinal discomfort, or other ill effects), replace it with another one.

### Supplemental Treatments
As a reinforcement effort for cleansing your liver, top off the herbal treatment with the following remedies:
- Sulfur trace element
- Hot-water bottle, once a day in the evening
- Reflexology massage, once or twice a day for five to fifteen minutes
- Supplements (brewer's yeast or bee pollen)
- Exercises/bends

## In Practice

- Based on your personal needs and the condition of your liver, you can opt for a simple or intensive treatment of varying duration, long or short. Combine the protocol you choose with other procedures for stimulating the liver (hepatic plants, hot-water bottle, exercises, massage, and so forth).

- For all these treatments, dietary reform is essential. At the very least, eliminate the most harmful foods.

# INDEX

# ABOUT THE AUTHOR

**www.christophervasey.ch**

Christopher Vasey, author and naturopath, practices his profession in Chamby-Montreux, Switzerland.

He pursued his studies at the naturopathy school in Paris under the guidance of Pierre-Valentin Marchesseau and Alain Rousseaux.

He opened his consulting office in 1979. In addition to his activities as a therapist, he continues to study natural medicine on his own in the books by the great naturopaths such as Dr. Paul Carton, Robert Masson, Herbert Shelton, and Dr. Edouard Bertholet.

In 1981 he began teaching introductory naturopathy to a wide range of health professionals. Since publishing his first book in 1988, he has been writing books on natural medicine for Éditions Jouvence, many of which have been translated into English by Healing Arts Press. These include *Natural Remedies for Inflammation, Optimal Detox, Freedom from Constipation,* and the best-selling *Acid-Alkaline Diet.* His books have also been translated into Chinese, German, Portuguese, Russian, Arabic, Chinese, and more.

Christopher Vasey lectures regularly in France, Switzerland, Belgium, Scandinavia, Iceland, Canada, and the United States.

# BOOKS OF RELATED INTEREST

**The Acid-Alkaline Diet for Optimum Health**
Restore Your Health by Creating pH Balance in Your Diet
*by Christopher Vasey, N.D.*

**Freedom from Constipation**
Natural Remedies for Digestive Health
*by Christopher Vasey, N.D.*

**Natural Remedies for Inflammation**
*by Christopher Vasey, N.D.*

**The Water Prescription**
For Health, Vitality, and Rejuvenation.
*by Christopher Vasey, N.D.*

**The High Blood Pressure Solution**
A Scientifically Proven Program for
Preventing Strokes and Heart Disease
*by Richard D. Moore, M.D., Ph.D.*

**Total Life Cleanse**
A 28-Day Program to Detoxify and Nourish the Body,
Mind, and Soul
*by Jonathan Glass, M.Ac., C.A.T.*

**Adaptogens**
Herbs for Strength, Stamina, and Stress Relief
*by David Winston and Steven Maimes*

**Candida Albicans**
Natural Remedies for Yeast Infection
*by Leon Chaitow, D.O., N.D.*

INNER TRADITIONS • BEAR & COMPANY
P.O. Box 388
Rochester, VT  05767
1-800-246-8648
www.InnerTraditions.com

Or contact your local bookseller